e-Health Technology: Concepts, Strategy, Exchange & Security

I0503646

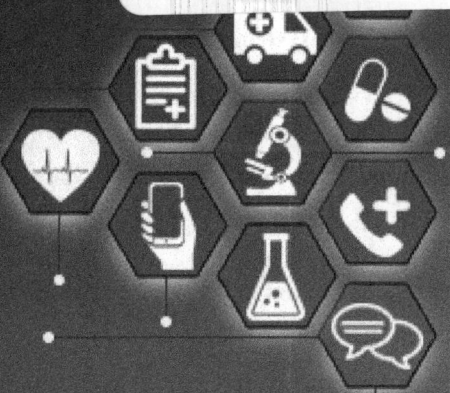

Rephael Akangbe &
Hosna Salmani

Published by: J-CUBE Hall

Tel: +2348028668951, +2348099888600

E-mail: raphelgloria@gmail.com

e-Health Technology: Concepts, Strategy, Exchange and Strategy Pocket Book @ 2020 by Raphael Akangbe and Hosna Salmani

For further information, enquiries, permission, please write us:

Raphael Akangbe raphelgloria@gmail.com, &

Hosna Salmni hosnasalmani@gmail.com, salmani.h@tak.iums.ac.ir

PREFACE

The overall aim of this handbook is to provide a practical guide on the understanding of eHealth technology. Over the years, we have seen a steady growth in the number and type of eHealth technology, being adopted in different healthcare settings. Proponents of these systems claim eHealth can improve the quality of care provided, leading to better provider performance and health outcomes. Yet the evidence for such claims is mixed thus far, with some studies demonstrating benefits, others showing little to no impact, and some settings being even worse off than before. Understandably, there are now increasing pressures on government agencies and health organizations to demonstrate tangible return on value for the significant eHealth investments made.

Despite the growing importance and need to evaluate eHealth technology, there are relatively few formal courses available from post-secondary educational institutions on how health information management, health information technology, supports eHealth technology studies. Most educational institutions that offer degree programs related to health information management research, administration and services would typically include eHealth technology as part of their health research methods or program evaluation courses. Of those that offer health informatics degree programs, only some have eHealth technology as a full self-contained course. For institutions that offer eHealth technology as either a course or a topic within a course, the choice of textbooks and reference materials can vary greatly depending on what is available and the preference of the instructors.

Brief Notes from The Authors

E-health evolved out of a need for improved documentation and tracking of patients' health and procedures performed on patients, particularly for reimbursement purposes, such as by insurance companies. Traditionally, health care providers kept paper records on the history and status of their patients. However, rising health care costs and technological advances encouraged the development of electronic tracking systems. As e-health technologies continued to be developed, the field of telemedicine, in which telecommunication technologies are used to provide health care remotely, emerged.

E-health makes use of a wide array of digital technologies. The Internet, for example, allows e-health users to communicate with health care professionals by e-mail, to access medical records, to research health information, and to engage in person-to-person exchange of text, audio, video, and other data. Interactive TV, also known as polycom, provides both audio and visual transfer of a variety of information between two or more individuals at two or more locations in real time. Kiosks, which are freestanding devices (usually computers), are used in e-health to provide interactive information to the user. Most information is provided through a series of interactive prompts on a touch screen. Kiosks can also be used to collect data and information from users. DVDs, USB flash drives, and other media are used to store data digitally. Many modern mobile devices are designed with personal computing and Internet capabilities and are compatible with downloadable applications (or apps) that allow users to instantly access health information. Many of the technologies employed in e-health are accessible to all users, including those with impairments such as blindness or deafness.

Dr. Raphael Akangbe (DBA, Ph.D) & Hosna Salmani

CONTENTS

Preface

A Note from the Author

Table of Content

Chapter Eight

Chapter Nine

CHAPTER ONE

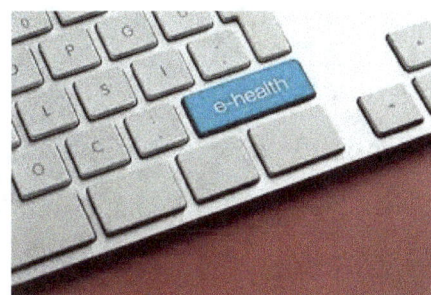

e-Health Information Technology

Introduction

The e-Health information provides unique security, privacy and confidentiality challenges that require a fresh examination of the mainstream concepts and approaches to information security. The importance of security and privacy in e-Health information raised the issues of individual consent, confidentiality and privacy, which are the main determinants in adopting and successful utilizing the e-Health information. Current trends in the domain of e-Health information management point to the need for comprehensive incorporation of security, privacy and confidentiality safeguards within the review of e-Health information management frameworks and approaches. This raises major challenges that demands holistic approaches spanning a wide variety of legal, ethical, psychological, information and security engineering. This introductory chapter explores information security and challenges facing e-Health information management.

The Trends and Nature of e-Health Information

The acceptability of Information Communication Technologies has created the electronic-health Information (e-Health Information) environment. At the core of e-Health is e-Health information, which is health information that is managed and delivered through ICTs. The major promises from e-Health include the lowering of costs, improvement of quality of patient care and enabling of better planning and decision-making. The delivery of these promises are hinged on e-Health's focus on the challenging goal of meeting the clinician's information requirements and enabling the integration of e-Health information with decision support systems and their delivery as on-line resources. However, the success of electronic Health-care will depend on whether it can ensure patient privacy, confidentiality and trust in managing e-health information.

The e-health information is varied and complex in nature. It is collected, maintained and utilized by a variety of players within the health-care profession as well as in other sectors, where it is required for purposes such as insurance, employment and research. The structure of health-care is multi-dimensional as it can be viewed in time-oriented, source-oriented and clinical problem-oriented terms **(Grimson, 2001)** with further dimensions being possible. In practice, health information is scattered across and within organizations and countries. The period for utilizing health information spans over a lifetime of an individual, i.e., from cradleto-grave, and even beyond. There may be a statutory time period from the death of a person after whose expiry the deceased's health-care information may be destroyed **(Lennon, 2005)**.

The destruction of health information by a controller of such information is a legally regulated process (Roach et al., 2006). A key aspect of the nature of health-care information is that it is personal. This perception has been recognized since the 4th Century BC at the inception of the medical profession through the Hippocratic Oath **(Baker and Masys, 1999)**.

It is recognised that health information belongs to the individual who is the subject of such information. The assertion that the health service provider owns health information while the law merely grants some interest and rights over the information to the patient is true for the USA **(Roach et al., 2006)**. It appears that this approach is increasingly being discarded in Europe, where it seems legal ownership of health information is bestowed on the patient while the health-care unit is designated as a controller with legal rights, interests and obligations over the information. Thus, use of health information always requires the consent of the individual owner.

In practice, there is a separation between ownership and control of health information, the owner of health information may not be the one who controls its collection, storage and processing. Therefore, this necessitates distinction between owners, the controllers, processors and users of health-care information **(Lennon, 2005)**. The later are governed by the laws on the protection of information to ensure the consent and preserve the owners' privacy and confidentiality.

In 2001, Grimson envisaged the next generation Electronic Health-care or Medical Records (EHR) as "a longitudinal cradle-to-the-grave active record readily accessible and available via the Internet to drive the delivery of health-care to the individual citizen" (Grimson, 2001). The attainment of such an EHR remains a future goal up to now.

In present practices, the EHRs are health information that is controlled and managed through ICTs. Thus, largely inaccessible to the individual control and use. While, Electronic Personal Health Records (EPHRs) **(Lafky and Horan, 2008)** are primarily health information that is directly controlled and managed through ICTs by the owner of the information, i.e., the individual who is the subject of the health information.

The individual is responsible for creating, maintaining and controlling access to the information. The content and nature of both the EHRs and EPHRs would react the complexity of health information and need not necessarily differ. In fact, the need for interoperability and information sharing and exchange between the EHRs and EPHRs is widely recognized. The concept behind the EHRs has been in existence since start of the medical practice profession in the form of paper-based medical records. However, the EPHRs are emergent concepts, that are not widely used. The universal adoption of EPHRs could be difficult, if not almost impossible, due to privacy and confidentiality concerns. Other negative factors for EPHR adoption include computer literacy, affordability, computing resources, time constraints on the individual and internet connectivity. These factors also vary with geographic location with Third World regions offering the most challenges.

Security Impact of e-Health Information System

The current drive towards patient-centred approaches and paradigms in healthcare practice places patient consent, security, privacy and confidentiality concerns at the core of e-Health information system challenges. At the local, national and international levels, information protection laws are acting as catalysts for privacy and confidentiality.

Generally speaking, health information is scattered and distributed into disparate domain-specific palace of information that exist within and between healthcare service providers. The EHRs promise to manage, to deliver and distribute computing environment based on

Internet Technologies. The introduction of wireless devices, sensor, network-enabled devices integration, interoperability, security and trust among and between the EHR systems are emerging as the key ingredients for successful management of e-Health information in this complex environment. The efforts directed to guarantee the information quality, privacy, confidentiality and easing complexity of e-Health information are focusing on standardization.

Security of e-Health Information

The extreme violations of health professional ethics and Code have triggered determined efforts to ensure strict adherence to privacy and confidentiality safeguards. The nature of personal health information requires individual rights to be focused on privacy and confidentiality of managing information.

The Electronic Health Records (EHRs), Electronic Patient Records (EPRs) and Electronic Medical Records (EMRs) provide the basis for e-Health services. The information in these records (containing patient health information) needs to be shared amongst multiple healthcare providers and healthcare professionals, but privacy issues have been a major inhibitor in the implementation of the EHRs, EMRs and EPRs systems. Information and communication technologies (ICTs) form the backbone for eHealth in delivering patient care services. The Internet offers affordable worldwide coverage, which makes it a favourable and popular platform for e-Health.

The health information and systems are sensitive and generally require a higher degree of security than information and systems in other domains. The legitimate uses of health data are contentious and the balance between legitimate uses of eHealth information, the right to privacy and confidentiality is elusive. Thus, there is an uneasiness on the part of the individual about the maintenance, utilisation and transmission of the EHRs by healthcare service providers. Hence, the emerging calls for individual persons' choice and discretion captured in opt-in and opt-out provisions in the laws and policies governing healthcare service providers.

The question of when it can be said that all security requirements for a given case have been attained and absolute assurance has been established is hard to resolve. We can measure only the degree of security requirement satisfaction rather than certainty.

The problem in measuring the latter is one of the major challenges to attaining secure e-Health information. The complex nature of the healthcare environment renders the security of e-Health information difficult to develop appropriate adaptable policy for securing individual patient EHRs. However, it is noted that the unique capability of e-Health to transgress all existing geo-political and other barriers is a complicating factor in securing e-Health information. The policy development initiatives continue to take place largely in an isolated manner and lacks convergence with other aspects of securing e-Health information.

Matters in e-Health Information Security

The emerging e-Health development and investment in national and organizational strategic visions and plans worldwide will no doubt pose a threat that will derail the plans for e-Health information security. The identification of the key matters in e-Health information security, privacy and confidentiality is crucial to the success of e-Health. The misleading and controversial concepts that exist within the domain of computer security and the cross-fertilisation between this domain and other domains such as healthcare, law and organisational policy. This is an issue that is compounded within e-Health environment as these concepts take on extra domain and technology-specific connotations. Inter-disciplinary standardization efforts that take a holistic approach could help in reducing this problem. On a serious note, the issues of sharing and interoperability have continued to dominate e-Health information management. From the legal perspective, this matter arises where one jurisdiction imposes the condition that health information can only be transmitted to jurisdictions that have same information protection laws.

CHAPTER TWO

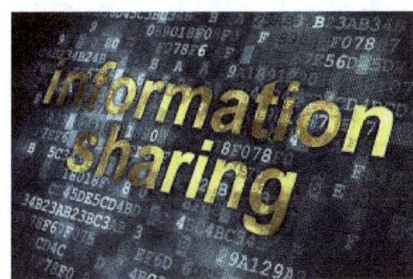

Information Sharing and Confidentiality

Introduction:

Information security and privacy in the health-care sector is an issue of growing importance. The adoption of digital patient records, increased regulation, provider consolidation and the increasing need for information exchange between patients, providers and payers, all point towards the need for better information security.

The technologies can help improve quality of health care delivery, the benefits of the technologies must be balanced with the privacy and security concerns of the user. Data from in-home sensors and medical records will be communicated electronically via the Internet and wireless transmissions. This increases the danger of compromising the security and privacy of individuals.

What is confidential patient information?

A duty of confidence arises when one person discloses information to another (e.g. patient to clinician) in circumstances where it is reasonable to expect that the information will be held in confidence. It is a legal obligation that is derived from case law and a requirement established within professional codes of conduct.

Patients entrust us with, or allow us to gather, sensitive information relating to their health and other matters as part of their seeking treatment. They do so in confidence and they have the legitimate expectation that staff will respect their privacy and act appropriately. In some circumstances patients may lack the competence to extend this trust, or may be unconscious, but this does not diminish the duty of confidence. It is essential, if the legal requirements are to be met and the trust of patients is to be retained, that the NHS provides, and is seen to provide, a confidential service. What this entails is described in more detail in subsequent sections of this document, but a key guiding principle is that a patient's health records are made by the health service to support that patient's healthcare.

One consequence of this is that information that can identify individual patients, must not be used or disclosed for purposes other than healthcare without the individual's explicit consent, some other legal basis, or where there is a robust public interest or legal justification to do so. In contrast, anonymize information is not confidential and may be used with relatively few constraints.

Patient information is generally held under legal and ethical obligations of confidentiality. Information provided in confidence should not be used or disclosed in a form that might identify a patient without his or her consent.

There are a number of important exceptions to this rule, described later in this document, but it applies in most circumstances.

Patient consent to disclosing

Patients generally have the right to object to the use and disclosure of confidential information that identifies them, and need to be made aware of this right. Sometimes, if patients choose to prohibit information being disclosed to other health professionals involved in providing care, it might mean that the care that can be provided is limited and, in extremely rare circumstances, that it is not possible to offer certain treatment options. Patients must be informed if their decisions about disclosure have implications for the provision of care or treatment. Clinicians cannot usually treat patients safely, nor provide continuity of care, without having relevant information about a patient's condition and medical history.

Where patients have been informed of:

a. the use and disclosure of their information associated with their healthcare; and

b. the choices that they have and the implications of choosing to limit how information may be used or shared.

The Confidentiality Model

The model outlines the requirements that must be met in order to provide patients with a confidential service. Record holders must inform patients of the intended use of their information, give them the choice to give or withhold their consent as well as protecting their identifiable information from unwarranted disclosures. These processes are inter-linked and should be ongoing to aid the improvement of a confidential service.

The four main requirements are:

a. Protect – look after the patient's information;

b. Inform – ensure that patients are aware of how their information is used;

c. Provide Choice – allow patients to decide whether their information can be disclosed or used in particular ways. To support these three requirements, there is a fourth:

d. Improve – always look for better ways to protect, inform, and provide choice.

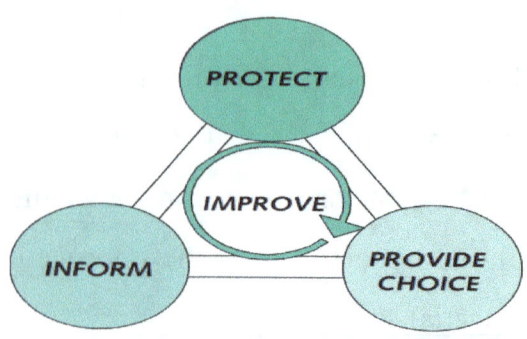

Confidentiality Model

Protect Patient Information

Patients' health information and their interests must be protected through a number of measures:

a. Procedures to ensure that all staff, contractors and volunteers are at all times fully aware of their responsibilities regarding confidentiality;

b. Recording patient information accurately and consistently;

c. Keeping patient information private;

d. Keeping patient information physically secure;

e. Disclosing and using information with appropriate care.

Security

The National Institute of Standards and Technology (NIST), the federal agency responsible for developing information security guidelines, defines information security as the preservation of data confidentiality, integrity, availability (commonly referred to as the "CIA" triad). Not only does the NIST provide guidance on securing data, but federal legislations such as the Health Insurance Portability and Accountability Act (HIPAA) and the Health Information Technology for Economic and

Clinical Health (HITECH) Act mandate doing so. Violating these regulations has serious consequences, including criminal and civil penalties for clinicians and organizations.

The increasing concern over the security of health information stems from the rise of EHRs, increased use of mobile devices such as the smart-phone, medical identity theft, and the widely anticipated exchange of data between and among organizations, clinicians, federal agencies, and patients. If patients' trust is undermined, they may not be forthright with the physician. For the patient to trust the clinician, records in the office must be protected. Medical staff must be aware of the security measures needed to protect their patient data and the data within their practices.

Data Access and Storage

There has long been concern over a patient's health record privacy and confidentiality. Connecting personal health information to the Internet exposes this data to more hostile attacks compared to the paper-based medical records.

Currently, patients have to physically go into a health care facility to get their medical record. Since the records are in paper format, this physically limits the number of people who see the record and how it gets transmitted. However, once this information is available electronically, it opens the way for hackers and other malicious attackers to access the records as well as those who are authorized. In addition, given the distributed nature of sensor networks for in-home patient monitoring, there is a greater challenge in ensuring data security and integrity compared to the traditional health care system. Eavesdropping and skimming are a possibility when the sensor data is transmitted wirelessly. Data access, storage, and integrity are key challenges when implementing EPRs and in-home sensor networks.

There are currently many different regulations and rules surrounding health care including the Federal Regulations of The American Health Insurance Portability and Accountability Act (HIPAA) as well as various state regulations.

While these regulations provide a framework of policy, they will have to be adapted as EPRs and sensors change the way health care is delivered. HIPAA is a set of rules to be followed by doctors, hospitals and other health care providers. HIPAA's goal is to ensure that all medical records, medical billing, and patient accounts meet certain consistent standards with regards to documentation, handling and privacy. Moreover, HIPAA requires that all patients be able to access their own medical records, correct errors or omissions, and be informed how their personal information is shared or used. Other provisions of HIPAA include notification of privacy procedures to the patients. At the same time, each state has specialized rules for how health care is handled, which are nicely described by the Health Privacy Project's The State of Health Privacy.

The Privacy Rule of HIPAA addresses the use

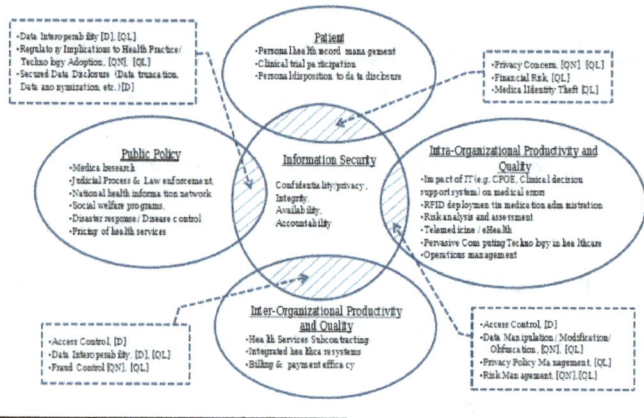

and disclosure of a patient's protected health information by healthcare plans, medical providers, and clearinghouses, also referred as "covered entities"

The Security Rule of HIPAA requires covered entities to ensure implementation of administrative safeguards in the form of policies and personnel, physical safeguards to information infrastructure, and technical safeguards to monitor and control intra and inter organizational information access.

Research Domains in the Healthcare Information Security

The issues of data access, storage, and analysis are not unique to the medical fields. These problems have been looked on in a number of areas, from financial services to internet shopping, and technical solutions exist which can be applied to health care to increase privacy and security in a multi-user setting:

• **Role-based access control**: one of the most challenging problems in managing large networks is the complexity of security administration. Role based access control, or role based security, is the dominant model for advanced access control. It results in the reduction of the complexity and cost of security administration in large networked applications.

• **Encryption:** Encryption can be used to ensure the security of the data and help prevent eavesdropping and skimming. Encryption can be accomplished in hardware as well as in software. In order to ensure the highest level of security, it is best if both forms of encryption are used. Different symmetric and asymmetric key algorithms can be used to provide encryption in software.

• **Authentication Mechanisms:** Authentication mechanisms can be used to ensure the data is coming from the person/entity. There has been a number of authentication algorithms developed such as passwords, digital signatures, and challenge response authentication protocol.

Data Interoperability and Information Security

Healthcare information systems currently adopted by some provider organizations store health information in different proprietary formats. This diversity of data formats creates a major hurdle in sharing patient data among provider organizations as well to medical and health policy research Healthcare information systems currently adopted by some provider organizations store health information in different proprietary formats. This diversity of data formats creates a major hurdle in sharing patient data among provider organizations as well to medical and health policy research. Investing in EMR interoperability and establishing a health information exchange, could save the industry $77B per year. Whereas without interoperability, continued adoption of current EMR technologies will promote information silos that already exist in today's paper based medical records leading to proprietary control by information creators. Moreover, privacy and security in establishing an interoperable health information exchange remain dominant issues. Recently, nationwide initiatives have been undertaken to address the privacy and security problems under the auspices of AHRQ and the Office of the National Coordinator for Health Information Technology. Currently 33 states and one territory have developed plans to implement privacy and security policy solutions that enable seamless electronic exchange of health information. Most of these state plans recognize the need and call for development of a universal patient consent form that incorporates common information disclosure situations as well for specially protected information. Furthermore they call for standardized approaches for user authorization and authentication, user access, and audit of patient record access and modification, uniform identification of patients, security of data during transmission and at rest. Development of fully functional interoperable EHR system remains a major challenge. Recent research has proposed prototype service-oriented architecture (SOA) models for EHR in various contexts including clinical decision support, collaborative medical (mammogram) image analysis, and health clinic setting. These SOA based EHRs are expected to be scalable to enable inter-enterprise environments such as regional health information organizations (RHIO), and alliance of such RHIOs could lead to national and global health information networks. In a case study based analysis of three emerging RHIOs, namely the Indian health Information Exchange, the Massachusetts Health Data Consortium, and the Santa Barbara County Care Data Exchange, Several factors that influence innovation and diffusion, adaptation, and change management of RHIOs are elicited. Among them, privacy and security of patient information are major concerns hampering the adoption of clinical information technologies across the RHIOs. Such concerns could remain in the near future as the technology standards for data interoperability are still in the development stage.

Health matrix

The perceived offense arises from expectations unique to the medical context. The expectations are not that information about one's medical problem won't be known or that one's intimate anatomy will not be physically exposed to others. Rather, it is that a patient expects that anyone who learns about medical problems or views intimate anatomy will be someone who must have that information in order to help. In other words, to the extent necessary for self-benefit, the patient consents to expose physical and medical information to direct care health care personnel but to no others. Other examples of common intrusions in daily medical encounters may be easily imagined: ancillary health care workers learn of medical details beyond their need to know; partially disrobed patients are placed on stretchers in hallways or behind half-drawn curtains; open patient charts are inadvertently left on nursing station countertops and are able to be read by others. But legal cases of this sort are virtually non-existent. In many cases, patients may not find out about such occurrences or, where they are aware, may consider the type of privacy such occurrences invade to be one they already expect to be compromised in the course of competent medical care. Even if they believe that "this shouldn't happen," patients are not likely to litigate the more mundane intrusions. The "publicity of private facts" tort seems like it should be a natural fit for unauthorized disclosures of medical information, but most cases fail if its elements are strictly applied. The requirements that the private information is "of no legitimate public interest" and that its disclosure would be "highly offensive" and likely to cause serious mental injury to a reasonable person of "ordinary sensibilities" may be satisfied in many situations, but the broad dissemination requirement poses an obstacle. Courts often struggle to determine how many persons must have learned of the private facts before reaching the threshold for liability.

In the medical context, denying a remedy on grounds that a disclosure is not public enough does not adequately take into account the unique nature of medical information or the structure of the encounter in which it is learned. While "private" information is commonly known by an intimate or small circle close to an individual, medical information is often much more sensitive. Medical information involves matters that often would not readily be known by any third party, even friends or intimate relations, absent disclosure by the patient himself. Details about bodily functions, concerns about sexual functioning or sexuality, a history of substance abuse, and battles with troubled thoughts are beyond the commonplace private sphere. Disclosing a highly sensitive private fact without authorization to even one person would then make it "public." Revelation of a diagnosis or prognosis to even a very limited audience may place people at risk of social isolation and very real, albeit illegal, discrimination. Furthermore, sharing medical information with third parties without authorization from the patient assaults an individual's dignity and may be wrongful even in the absence of proof of further damages.

Confidentiality is fundamental to the trust upon which the doctor-patient relationship is founded. A doctor has a duty to respect patient confidentiality because:

(i) Information about a person's health is private;

(ii) a patient's willingness to provide information of relevance to diagnosis and treatment is founded on a guarantee of confidentiality

Confidentiality and privacy concerns related to health care long predate the implementation of HIPAA. The types of concerns patients express may be sorted into categories. Non-physicians were more commonly associated with privacy related complaints than were attending or resident physicians.

Patient Confidentiality

Ensuring the security, privacy and protection of patient healthcare data is critical for all healthcare personnel and institutions. In this age of fast-evolving information technology, this is truer than ever before. In the past, healthcare workers often collected patient data for research and usually only omitted the patients' names. This is no longer permitted, now any protected health information (PHI) that can identify a patient or the patient's relatives, employers, or household members, must be omitted before being used for research. The Health Insurance Portability and Accountability Act (HIPAA) Public Law, was enacted into federal law to ensure that that patient medical data remains private and secure. There are two main sections of the law, the Privacy Rule which address the use and disclosure of individuals' health information and the Security Rule which sets national standards for protecting the confidentiality, integrity, and availability of electronic protected health information. The Privacy Rule specifies 18 elements that constitute PHI. These identifiers include demographic and other information relating to the past, present, or future physical or mental health or condition of an individual, or the provision or payment of health care to an individual.

HIPPA was enacted to encompass three areas of patient care:

1. Portability of insurance or the ability of a patient/worker to move to another place of work and be certain that insurance coverage is not denied

2. Detection and enforcement of fraud and accountability

3. Simplify administrative procedures in health care and other professions (this is an area where communication and transmission of records are done electronically).

The penalties for failing to comply with HIPAA can be severe.

To whom does HIPAA apply?

HIPAA applies to all healthcare institutions and healthcare workers, who submit claims electronically. For example, if you are a healthcare worker and transmit or even discuss PHI with others who are not involved with that patient's care, then you violate HIPAA. However, there is a HIPAA rule that permits disclosure of PHI without prior obtained consent for healthcare operations, treatment, and payment. This includes consultation between providers regarding a patient, referring a patient and information required by law for public health safety and reporting. These exceptions cover the majority of clinical uses of PHI. Other disclosures demand explicit patient consent and apply to everyone in a healthcare facility, including:

- Doctors

- Nurses

- Pharmacists

- Administrative personnel

- Foodservice

- Clerical

- Janitorial service

- All other healthcare professionals

The HIPAA policies also apply to any interns and volunteers who work under supervision at a health clinic or hospital, third-party contractors or business associates, including:

- External laboratories

- External imaging services

- Outside computer repairman

- Accredited agencies that conduct patient surveys

- Medical equipment companies

- Pharmaceutical salespeople

Definition of PHI

HIPAA broadly defines PHI as any health information that is transmitted or maintained in electronic media. It is also important to know that PHI is not only restricted to electronic transmission of media, but also any oral communications of individually identifiable health information constitutes PHI. For example, if a surgery resident speaks about a surgical procedure in an elevator full of people that can be a HIPAA violation if any PHI is mentioned. The majority of medical records in healthcare institutions and clinics meet the definition of PHI, some of which include:

- Admission profile
- Billing records

- Patient profile
- Prescription records
- Referrals
- Discharge and follow up appointments

Hence all healthcare institutions and clinics must satisfy HIPAA standards for security and privacy.

Specific HIPAA Rules That Pertain to PHI Security

1. Ensure that there is integrity, confidentiality, and security of all electronic PHI that the healthcare institution creates, maintains, receives or transmits

2. Develop protection against any reasonably anticipated hazards or threats

to the integrity of the security of such data

3. Protect against any reasonably anticipated use or disclosure of information that is not permitted or required

4. Ensure compliance among the workforce

5. Have flexibility in the system, so patient care is not compromised

6. Covered entities may use any security that meets the minimal standards

7. The type of security depends on the size, complexity, and capabilities of the covered entity

Patient Rights under HIPAA

HIPAA rules give patients' rights, some of which they may not be not aware. The most important rights of patients under HIPAA include the following:

Right to receive a Notice of Privacy Practices

- Right to restrict PHI disclosures
- Right to state how they want PHI to be handled and communicated to others. For example, the patient may want any message from the pharmacist or the hospital to be sent by mail to his private home and not left on his home phone number
- Right to inspect and review their PHI. If the patient perceives there to be anything erroneous in the PHI, they do have the

right to request a change. The provider may accept or deny this request. For example, a nurse may have been diagnosed with bipolar disorder and after treatment may want this diagnosis to be deleted from the medical chart. This is not a request that can be accepted.

- Right to obtain a copy of their PHI
- Right to receive an accounting of where PHI disclosures have been made
- The right to report to the Office of Civil Rights if the patient believes there has been any violation of disclosure

Sharing confidential patient information

The NHS Constitution explains that patients have the right to privacy and confidentiality, the right to expect the NHS to keep patient confidential information safe and secure, and the right to be informed about how their information is used.

Patients also have the right to request that their confidential information is not used beyond their own care and treatment, to have their objections considered, and, where their wishes cannot be followed, to be told the reasons including the legal basis.

Policies on confidential patient data seek to strike a balance between the protection of patient information, and the use and sharing of information to improve care, such as for research purposes.

Patient information that is kept by health and social care providers must be securely safeguarded. Patient-doctor confidentiality is considered one of the cornerstones of medical practice. The BMA's Confidentiality and disclosure of health information tool kit states that:

Confidentiality is an essential requirement for the preservation of trust between patients and health professionals and is subject to legal and ethical safeguards. Patients should be able to expect that information about their health which they give in confidence will be kept confidential unless there is a compelling reason why it should not.

The sharing of anonymised patient information more widely can potentially bring about improvements to patient care. For example, tracking and analysis of patient health information can help with medical research and with the design of more effective services. Information used in this way must be anonymised and untraceable to individuals before it is released for this purpose. NHS Digital is responsible for ensuring that data is suitable for being used in this way.

Privacy and security in Healthcare:

Confidentiality and privacy refer to how professionals must handle pieces of information gathered during medical care. Confidentiality concerns the attitude required of professionals to handle information resulting from this relationship. The three attributes – secrecy, privacy and confidentiality – are professional obligations when handling information. In addition, these three attribute are also rights of users.

Primary health care teams, which also include community health agents, access and handle a lot of information on users. Thus, it is appropriate to discuss how to respect the secrecy and privacy of such information while working in a multidisciplinary team. The exchange of information between users and professionals is, in principle, related to the trust created in their relationship.

Ensuring the privacy, security, and confidentiality of personal health information has been a fundamental principle for the health information management (HIM) profession throughout its 80-year history. Today, HIM professionals continue to face the challenge of maintaining the privacy and security of patient information, an effort that grows in complexity as information becomes more and more distributed in electronic systems. The challenge of this responsibility has also increased due to the constantly changing legislative and regulatory environment.

Regulations have impacted privacy and security:

- The Health Insurance Portability and Accountability Act of 1996 (HIPAA)

- The American Recovery and Reinvestment Act of 2009 (ARRA)
- Modifications to the HIPAA Privacy, Security, and Enforcement Rules the Health Information Technology for Economic and Clinical Health Act; Final Rule

Privacy and security are critical success factors in the movement toward EHR adoption. As the industry continues to change, the HIM professional is positioned to grow in the role of privacy and security advocate. HIM professionals who serve in this advocacy function are diverse, including organizational and corporate privacy officers, compliance officers, change agents in policy development, advocates for privacy and security assurances as EHR systems are implemented and demands for information become more diverse, and representatives for consumers who often distrust the systems that house their most sacred medical stories.

Privacy Rule:

The Privacy Rule sets the floor providing baseline requirements to preserve the overall confidentiality of protected health information (PHI) regardless of type (e.g. verbal, paper, electronic).

- Protects individuals' health records and other individually identifiable health information created, maintained, or received by or on behalf of covered entities and their business associates

- Protects individuals' PHI by regulating the circumstances under which covered entities may use and disclose protected health information

- Covered entities are required to have contracts or other arrangements in place with business associates that perform functions for or provide services to, or on behalf of, the covered entity

- Gives individuals rights with respect to their protected health information, including rights to examine and obtain a copy of their health records and to request corrections

Security Rule:

The Security Rule applies only to protected health information in electronic form

- Requires covered entities to implement certain administrative, physical, and technical safeguards to protect electronic information
- Covered entities have contracts in place with their business associates that all business associates will appropriately safeguard the electronic protected health information they receive, create, maintain, or transmit on behalf of the covered entities

CHAPTER THREE

Personal e-Health Information Protection

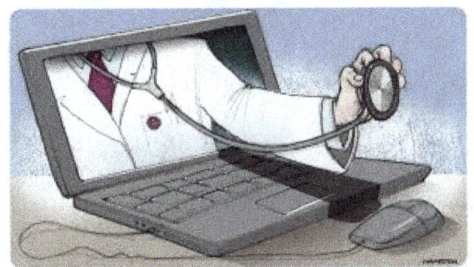

Introduction

Protecting personal e-Health information aims mainly at securing the privacy and confidentiality of the individual who receives healthcare services that are delivered through e-Health. Advances in security technologies have so far not eliminated the challenge posed by the need to secure e-Health information. The rate of privacy and confidentiality breaches continue to increase unabated. These breaches pose challenges to all domains that converge on the task of securing information and building trust in e-Health information management. Only a holistic approach that positions itself at the point of convergence of the domains of law, organizational policy, professional ethics and IT security could offer the promise to mitigate, if not eliminate, the major challenges to securing e-Health information. As efforts to digitize information are swiping across nearly all walks of life, healthcare providers are faced with a problem of protecting patients' privacy. While this is not a new problem, it is more difficult to protect patients' privacy in e-Health due to sensitive and complex nature of the information to be protected and the increasingly sophisticated environment in which the protection is to operate. The e-Health information management is a domain in which pro-actively securing and safeguarding the privacy of individual healthcare information is of fundamental importance. Several techniques have been devised to protect data such as encryption, digital signatures and anonymization. By using these techniques healthcare providers become more competitive, trustworthy and increase use of e-Health information systems. Healthcare service organizations that maintain e-Health information systems are entrusted with the responsibility and duty to manage personal health information held in these systems. Thus, securing e-Health information is a growing and on-going concern.

This chapter explores the main impediments in securing e-Health information and the nature and theory of secure e-Health information.

Violations of Privacy and Confidentiality in e-Health Information

The ever-growing catalogue of personal privacy and confidentiality breaches is posing major challenges as more and more healthcare organisations embrace e-Health and computerize their healthcare information management processes. Some of these violations are accidental, while others are the result of ethically questionable actions undertaken by business organisations, or a general laxity in securing sensitive e-Health information that is controlled by the organisation. The data security includes both confidentiality and integrity. The confidentiality is required to keep sensitive information from being disclosed to unauthorised individuals, while integrity can be explained as having the data in the information system totally accurate and consistent. Privacy and confidentiality are two terms that have been considered synonymous and used interchangeably within the healthcare community.

Information Technology Security Challenge for Protecting e-Health Information

The IT safety focuses mainly on the protection of security and integrity of information and the prevention of information theft. Thus, systematic attempts are made and appropriate technical safeguards are mounted to prevent data loss anyhow and unauthorized individuals from inappropriately obtaining information in general without regard to domain-specific nuances. The major IT security challenges lies in the following areas:

1. authentication and authorization;

2. security certification;

3. data security focusing on cryptography and;

4. integrity and non-repudiation.

The advances in computer storage, networking and information processing technologies have enabled increasingly massive collections of electronic data. Ability to communicate and process such data at high speed and access it remotely is a cause for security, privacy and confidentiality concerns. These concerns are further complicated by the existence of methods and technologies of analyzing such data. In particular, data mining promises to efficiently discover valuable information and knowledge from massive electronic information sources. Thus, data mining is particularly vulnerable to misuse in breaching security, privacy and confidentiality. The desire for the protection of the ownership and privacy of individual e-Health information without impeding information flow during healthcare service delivery points to a challenge for the database community to design information systems that offer adequate protection **(Agrawal et al., 2003).**

The e-Health distributed environment takes the issue of access control well beyond geographical locations. The shared care paradigm brings in many players and roles along an extended geographical dimension with the context of patient care. This complicates access control and creates risks of violations. Presently, consensus has been reached that the patient owns personal e-Health information. The existing irony is that the patient has no access control over personal e-Health information held in the systems.

Privacy and Confidentiality Issues

The privacy issues that are involved provide individuals with the ability to control how their e-Health information should be managed and used by clinicians as well as other users in domains other than healthcare. Privacy is usually protected by the law, which imposes a duty on designated entities and systems to ensure that individuals are able to exercise their privacy rights. Privacy and confidentiality within the healthcare community are so closely related that the two have come to be considered as one and the same and are sometimes used interchangeably. Thus, Anderson observed that other authors view confidentiality as protecting the interest of the organisation and privacy as protecting the autonomy of the individual while privacy and confidentiality means the same in common medical usage **(Anderson and Cardell, 2008).** Although *e-Health confidentiality governs the disclosure of* *personal healthcare information, but privacy grants a right to control disclosure to the individual patient while confidentiality imposes a duty on healthcare providers not to disclose the information and to ensure that individual patient exercise their privacy rights in controlling circumstances where they will allow disclosure by healthcare providers to happen.* Thus, it would seem, from this distinction of the two terms, that while *privacy is an individual's right, confidentiality is an obligation on trusted professionals and organisations to protect privacy and the exercise of the rights, it grants to the individual.*

The major challenges arise from the fact that, on one hand, in practice, the individual is generally not in a strong position to control disclosure of personal eHealth information, while, on the other hand, confidentiality within e-Health is at risk under a multiplicity of threats occasioned by technological advances and organizational factors. The area of prescription data collection, processing and mining provides a typical example of a domain where, in practice, the patient currently is in a weak position to control the disclosure of their prescription-related information **(Cook, 2007)**. This will remain so until certain conditions and developments occur within the e-Health information management domain.

One such major development is the wide adoption of the electronic personal health record

(EPHR) by the individual, who will have full control. This will need to be accompanied by official recognition of EPHRs for use during daily patient care practice. Another major development would be the emergence of wholistic and comprehensive frameworks and their implementations for securing e-Health information in a way that takes into account the information protection laws, security and healthcare record standards, appropriate computer security methods and technologies The rapid evolution of e-Health has a huge impact on the protection of patient information. Furthermore, the e-Health environment has the capacity to facilitate rapid, massive, and potentially undetected violations of patient privacy and confidentiality. Juxtaposing these potentialilties of e-Health with the public concerns about privacy and confidentiality has led to the recognition by professional and state bodies that the protection of information given to healthcare providers is a fundamental ethical obligation to all healthcare professions.

The fact that the patient gives the information to healthcare providers in confidence and out of necessity is a key factor that sums ethical and moral dimensions to the health information management activities of those in control of personal health information. Protecting the privacy of patients' identifiable health information is a significant issue for the success of e-Health and realization of its promises.

The patients disclose information to healthcare providers out of necessity to obtain treatment and improve their health. This information is given in-confidence. The patients' understanding is that the primary purpose for the disclosure, collection and storage of personal healthcare information is for their current and future medical care. When such personal healthcare information is used for other purposes that have nothing to do with their healthcare, it becomes a matter of serious privacy and confidentiality concern.

The Government has invoked the common good to justify secondary uses of personal e-Health information in activities that aimed at benefiting society as a whole. However, it is questionable whether profit motives in the secondary uses of personal e-Health information is justifiable or not.

At a national level, personal health information is important for use in computing vital statistics that are needed in planning and resource allocation. Furthermore,the national control of infectious and epidemic diseases largely involve close scrutiny and disclosure of personal health information outside the patient care domain. The legal protection of personal privacy and confidentiality is of crucial significance to the advancement of democracy at a national level.

Critical View of The Utilisation Challenges of e-health Information

The multi-purpose use of e-Health information has given rise to chronic challenges for securing e-Health information. The e-Health information is personal and its primary purpose is to aid in decision-making of clinical care of an identified individual. Thus, for primary use purposes, the correct and accurate identification of individual subject of healthcare information is of fundamental importance.

Furthermore, the individual and the information benefit privacy and confidentiality protection from both medical professional ethics and the law. Other uses of e-Health information are referred to as secondary uses.

The veil of protection essentially precludes secondary purposes or uses of personal health information, which help in the management of diseases outbreaks. The secondary uses of health information can be viewed as a trade-off between individual privacy and society's necessity to reduce healthcare costs and improve quality and efficiency of the healthcare service. It is necessary to use the EHRs in clinical or epidemiological research, assessment of care quality and healthcare service planning and management. Therefore, the secondary uses of e-Health information have led to enhance patients' benefits through a well-managed healthcare service. Any secondary use of e-Health information, whether it does or does not bring benefits to the individual or the public, e.g., the use of information to deny employment or health insurance, gives rise to privacy and confidentiality concerns as well as legal and ethical considerations. Ethical considerations are managed through the various healthcare professions.

Insight To Legal Protection Challenges

The challenges that occur at the boundary of the law and utilisation of e-Health information for research purposes is the conflict between technical security on one hand and consent on the other hand. Technical security of health information may receive undue priority over consent in the e-Health information collection. Arnason **(Arnason, 2004)** decries that where the issue of consent enjoys priority, it has often appeared in confidential form, i.e., the demand for informed consent before participation in research. This has led Arnason **(Arnason, 2004)** to propose an alternative replacement for consent or presumed consent, which requires written authorisation based on general information to be used in research.

The challenges in the legal protection of e-Health information relate to the enforcement and mandate of data protection agencies. In many countries the data protection is very weak. Therefore, incentive for industries and public bodies to incorporate privacy principles into their IT systems and services should be encouraged **(EPTA, 2006)**.

Nature of Secure e-Health Information

The nature of secure e-Health information is characterized in terms of security, privacy and confidentiality requirements from the domain of healthcare as well as the legal protections. The principles for personal information held in a database that proclaim to be Hippocratic **(Agrawal et al., 2002)** clearly express one proposal for the key elements of the secure management of e-Health information.

An attractive feature of these principles is their derivation from the law, guidelines and policy for the healthcare domain. An implementation of these principles as proposed for Hippocratic databases represents a convergence of law and technology for securing e-Health information.

The ten principles were presented by Agrawal **(Agrawal et al., 2002)** and can be expressed within the context of e-Health information management as follows:

1. The purpose for which an individual's e-Health information has been collected shall be associated with that information (purpose specification);

2. The purposes associated with personal e-Health information shall have the consent of the donor of the information (consent);

3. The e-Health information collected shall be limited to the minimum necessary for accomplishing the specified purpose (limited collection);

4. The e-Health information shall be subjected to only those queries that are consistent with the purpose for which the information has been collected (limited use);

5. The e-Health information shall not be communicated outside the database for purposes other than those for which there is consent from the donor/owner of the information (limited disclosure);

6. The e-Health information shall be retained only as long as necessary for the fulfillment of the purpose for which it has been collected (limited retention);

7. The e-Health information about an individual shall be accurate and up-todate (accuracy);

8. Personal e-Health information shall be protected by security safeguards against theft and other forms of appropriation (safety);

9. An individual or a patient shall be able to access all e-Health information about himself or herself (openness); and

10. The donor/owner of e-Health information shall be able to verify compliance with these principles.

Similarly, an e-Health information system shall be able to address a challenge concerning compliance. The modern adoption of the shared care paradigm in healthcare necessitates the need to share e-Health information.

The technical solution to supporting sharing e-Health information is the interoperability between e-Health information systems.

It has been suggested that information exchange, supported by computable interoperability, is the key to many of the initiatives in e-Healt **(Orlova et al., 2005).** The openEHR community has recognized two forms of interoperability: syntactic interoperability and semantic interpretability. It has been suggested that semantic interoperability is a key requirement to enable the EHRs operations. The openEHR Foundation's archetype approach enables syntactic interoperability and semantic interpretability **(Garde S, 2007).**

The Fundamentals for Securing e-Healthcare Information

The main concepts for e-Health information security are reviewed. The objective is to formalise the theory of security, privacy, trust and confidentiality from the point of view of applications in e-Health Information Management. A more formal and clear distinction is drawn among the key concepts of security, privacy, confidentiality and trust. The security challenges posed by the presence or absence of individual Unique Identifier in e-Health information management is investigated as part of the theory. Privacy is the right to freely control the disclosure of personal e-

Health information **(RindÀeisch, 1997)** in a democratic society.

The right to privacy protects the autonomy of the individual with respect to controlling access to personal e-Health information. The key fields, that affect privacy, are security, access to information and services, societal interaction, convenience and economic benefit **(EPTA, 2006)**. These fields are evolving and hence subject to rapid change. Since the Internet lies at the core of e-Health, IT security is now recognised to be of key significance in e-Health, although the fight for the protection of patient privacy and confidentiality would seem new in e-Health information management.

The security principles that are promulgated by the International Information Security Foundation are:

• **Accountability principle** - information is not disclosed to unauthorised persons or processes;

• **Awareness principle** - owners, providers and users of information systems should easily be able to gain knowledge of and information about the existence and extent of security measures, practices and procedures;

• **Ethics principle** - the security of information should be provided in such a way that respects the rights and legitimate interest of others;

• **Multi-Disciplinary Principle** - security measures, practices and procedures should consider and address all issues and viewpoints including technical, administrative, organisational, operational, commercial, educational and legal aspects;

• **Proportionality Principle** - the overall investment and resource allocation to security should be proportionate and appropriate to the value and degree of reliance on the IT system and to severity, probability and extent of potential harm envisaged;

• **Integration Principle** - security measures should be coordinated and integrated with each other as well as with other organisational measures on other areas so as to create a coherent security system;

• **Timeliness Principle** - all parties at all levels should act in a timely manner in preventing and responding to security breaches;

• **Re-Assessment Principle** - security risk assessments should be carried out periodically as security requirements vary with time;

• **Equity Principle** - security of IT systems should be compatible with legal use and flow of data and information in a democracy.

Without doubt, the challenges facing e-Health include the following threats: *viruses*, *Trojans*, *worms causing denial-of-service attacks*, *impersonation*, *information theft*, *insiders privileged access to network operations and a grudge against their employer*. IT security is never absolute and measures can only be mitigatory. These measures include policies, procedures and employment of technology as well as performing information risk assessments and can be classified into administrative, physical and technical with legal and standards compliance falling into administrative measures. The main aspects that should be covered by IT security within e-Health are based on the following generic factors:

1. authentication, authorisation

2. security certification;

3. data security focusing on cryptography and;

4. integrity and non-repudiation.

Secure databases could play a key role in realising secure e-Health information. The same could be said for the use of e-privacy policies to formally specify a healthcare organisation's e-Health information management practices using XML-based policy definition language such as P3P *(platform for privacy policy preferences)* and EPAL *(enterprise privacy authorisation language)*.

The e-privacy policies could also formally specify an individual's privacy and confidentiality preferences. The alignment of privacy laws and organisational privacy policies to individual privacy concerns could be addressed by matching an organisation's privacy policy with individual's privacy preferences for health information access and use.

Since most e-Health information is held in databases, an interesting technological intervention is required that will enable database queries to automatically be modified, through query re-writing, that will conform to combined privacy scheme based on both privacy policy and user's privacy preferences.

Generally speaking, e-Health is not possible without distributed computing systems, because shared Care is the core paradigm for e-Health.

At the centre of the shared care paradigm is a model of patient care that envisages a healthcare service that is delivered by different clinicians, organisations, times and locations, using appropriate methods and tools that allow patient mobility.

The e-Health records (EHRs) form the informational foundation of communication and cooperation while a distributed computing infrastructure forms the technological foundation for such a complex shared care paradigm. Security within the distributed computing infrastructure for e-Health is complex, as it extends beyond both physical and conceptual domains in healthcare. It is further complicated by the sensitivity of personal e-Health information and must provide strong mutual authentication and accountability between communicating entities. While applications security is the second arm of distributed system security, it must provide services for accountability, authorisation and access control for information and functions.

Amalgamating Security with Privacy and Confidentiality

The extended nature of security domain in e-Health-supported shared care makes it impractical to grant authorisation for access to the EHRs on an individual basis. Privacy is the source of requirements, while IT security enables the realisation of these requirements. Therefore, there has to be a deliberate and targeted effort to ensure that patient privacy and confidentiality based on prevailing organisational policies and laws are implemented by means of IT security engineering. Confidentiality is enabled when IT security and privacy are combined. In other words, privacy and security is based on e-

Health management of confidentiality. Thus, it is possible for e-Health information systems to offer elements of IT security without protecting patient privacy and confidentiality.

It should be noted that privacy has been well established in the healthcare domain much longer than IT security. Shoniregun **(Shoniregun et al., 2004)** has explored how to be effective in managing customer relationship and advocated trust-based approach to viewing e-CRM.

Their research work demonstrated the organisational value of e-CRM and trust in eC within a multinational organisation and proposed the eC trust model, which incorporates people trust, technology trust and law and policy trust. These elements are also directly relevant as components of an e-Health trust model. The question *Shoniregun et al* posed can be mapped into the e-Health domain as:

How can e-Health information systems improve healthcare quality through information sharing and interoperability in a patient-centred managed care set-up while also securing higher level of patient trust on e-Health information management?

The public assessment of trust tends to address the views of patient care at the grass-root level. Policy makers who are concerned with the erosion of public trust need to target aspects associated with patient-centred care and professional expertise *(Calnan and Sanford, 2004)*, as these impact patient care quality. It has been noted that quality and trust are intertwined yet distinct concepts and their relation is not always straightforward *(Lampe et al., 2003)*.

Trust is generally a function of perceived quality, which in turn is a function of perceived professional expertise among other factors. Trust in physicians and medical institutions has been investigated in terms of what it is, whether is can be measured and whether it does matter *(Hall et al., 2001)*. The significance of trust is also illustrated by efforts that explore the relationship between continuity, trust in regular doctors and patient satisfaction with consultations with family doctors *(Baker et al., 2003)*. Thus, problems that are encountered in the ambulatory settings are found to be strongly related to lower trust *(Keating et al., 2002)*. Also elements of trust in hospitals have been found to include vulnerability to financial loss as well as expectations of competence and, hence, patient care quality *(Goold and Klipp, 2002)*.

Trust is a basis for an alternative care quality-enhancing approach suggested by Davies et al *(Davies and Lampel, 1998)*, which involves fostering greater trust in professionalism as a basis for quality enhancements instead of counter-productive mandatory publication of health outcomes. Therefore, Keating concluded that efforts to improve patients' experiences may promote more trusting relationships and greater continuity and should be a priority for physicians, educators, and health care organizations *(Keating et al., 2002)*.

Recognizing Securing e-Health Information

In many countries, frustration has been expressed based on the difficulties encountered in coordinating multiple sources of e-Health information in the absence of a unique personal recognition.

The ability to breach individual privacy and confidentiality has caused major concerns especially when modern data analysis and mining techniques are used as tools for this purpose. The universal personal identifier (UPI), anonymisation and pseudonymisation are emerging concepts that impact the security of e-Health information. Unresolved problem in e-Health is how the widely proposed standardize nationwide EHR system would uniquely identify and match a distributed composite of an individual's recorded healthcare information to a recognized individual patient out of approximately 300 million people to a 1:1 match *(Leonard, 2008)*.

Integrating systems without a reliable unique personal identifier (UPI) in many countries *(Grimson et al., 2000)* and between health (person-based records) and social care (care-based records-e.g. child protection) has been singled out as one of the major challenges for using routinely collected primary care data in e-Health and research *(de Lusignan and van Weel, 2006)*. Arellano and Weber *(Arellano and Weber, 1998)* paint a particularly grim picture of this problem.

The absence of a UPI has also been associated with problems of identifying potential participants for trial, access to records to confirm events, continued follow-up of patients during and after the trial, and secondary use of the trial data *(Armitage et al, 2008)*.

The advantage of the UPI is to enable a model, whereby Electronic Health Records (EHRs) are stored on a remote central server. The EHRs can be accessed by doctors using a smart-card, which contains unique identifiers that facilitate secured, remote, transportable access by consulting physicians at the discretion of the patient *(Dalley et al., 2006)*. The major disadvantage of the absence of the UPI is that patients' identities may not be reconcilable across institutions, and individuals with records held in different institutions will be falsely "counted" as multiple persons when databases are merged *(Berman, 2004)*.

The major concern with UPIs is privacy and confidentiality risks. If the UPI gets into the hands of the third party, it will create a severe security risk. The possible solution for reducing the UPI security risks is the Master Patient Index (MPI) file *(Freriks, 2000)*. Even though anonymisation and pseudonymisation are used to remove personally identifiable information, it is not enough to preserve the data confidentiality *(Chiang et al., 2003).*

The need for Universal Identifier in e-Health is best illustrated by the French Personal Medical Record (PMR), which has raised many important questions regarding duplicates and the quality, precision and coherence of the linkage with other health data coming from different sources. The currently planned identifying process in the French ministry of Health raises questions with regards to its ability to deal with potential duplicates and to perform data linkage with other health data sources. Using the electronic health records, Quantin et al developed and proposed an identification process to improve the French PMR *(Quantin et al., 2007)*.

Assessment of Anonymisation and Pseudonymisation

The near complete removal of the PII from the EHRs is achieved either through anonymisation or pseudonymisation. These two concepts are introduced in this subsection.

The problem and approaches to solutions for e-Health information anonymization and pseudonymisation are discussed:

(a) Anonymisation Anonymisation (which is also called sanitization or de-identification) is a result of the need to share or exchange information because of the business, standards or regulatory requirements. Anonymisation promotes information sharing and shared analysis among trusted or untrusted parties, while making sure that the probability of being able to make inference on personal identified information is low.

The essence of anonymisation is to hide private information, promote sharing, analysis and foster trust from individuals whose data is being anonymised. The anonymised data is useful in a number of applications such as healthcare research, business marketing campaigns and information exchange between organisations in the same market segment or across multiple organisations. We are currently witnessing generation, collection, storage and shared analysis (in some cases we need restricted analysis) of a huge amount of data worldwide.

There are cases where information must be stored without allowing any modification (e.g. information on the taxes) in such a case data encryption and access policies are one of the ways to protect data. There are situations where information can be altered in order to protect the privacy of the data owners (e.g. medical data can be modified previous to their release, so that researchers are able to study the data without jeopardising the privacy of patients).

The main challenge in the latter case is the problem on how data can be modified to minimise or prevent the possibility of information inference, thus guaranteeing the privacy of individuals. The anonymisation is used to remove or obfuscate any identifying information about a patient in a data set, making the re-identification or inference of an individual very difficult. In other words, the data should be shareable by adhering to privacy (what you cannot reveal) and analysis (what you must reveal) constraints. Data anonymisation can be applied to collection, retention and disclosure in a healthcare environment.

Data anonymisation is a long term problem. Therefore, before applying any of the techniques, a thorough *threat analysis* must be carried out. This is important, because what we want to protect today may not be what we may need to hide in the future. It is important to understand the trade-off of anonymisation and threat modelling not only from scientific and engineering point of view, but from society. The need for sharing personal data play a crucial role in driving anonymisation efforts.

Microsoft and Google both agreed to be part of the Networking Advertising Initiative that provides the data anonymisation. Customers in healthcare environment expect free, convenient and private way in which their vital e-Health information is maintained. It is important to note that even when data is anonymised, there is always a possibility of being able to infer on personal information. Therefore, the optimal solution for anonymity is difficult (currently only heuristic solutions is possible). Some of the lingering questions in the area of anonymisation are: *Is there any need to anonymise data that is stored? Do we just need secure storage using encryption? Are there any best practices in anonymisation? And is this just a research exercise?*

(b) Pseudonymisation We have noted that anonymisation removes PII *(Personally Identifiable Information)* of the individual from the EHRs mainly because the identity of the individual is not required for secondary use of the EHRs. However, situations exist where it may be required to re-create the link between the EHR and the individual to which the EHR belongs *(Iacono, 2007)*. Such situations include handling follow-up data, individual's request to withdraw their information, further treatment of a patient in light of new discoveries and quality control.

Maintaining privacy while allowing such re-identification of the individual is achieved through pseudonymisation. Neubauer and Riedl *(Neubauer and Riedl, 2008)* define the concept of pseudonymisation as:

a technique where identification data is transformed into, and afterwards replaced by, a specifier, which cannot be associated with the identification data without knowing a certain secret.

The pseudonymisation allows re-identification of the individual associated with an EHR subject. This involves the identification and separation of personal data from other data in the EHRs. Riedl *(Riedl et al., 2008)* considers de-personalisation of EHRs as a process that precedes and is necessary for pseudonymisation. Iacono *(Iacono, 2007)* identifies two pseudonymisation schemes that are based on the ability to be reversible. The first is the one-way pseudonymisation scheme, which generate pseudonyms which are impossible to be used to re-identify the patients. This type of scheme requires the maintenance of a mapping database to store associations between pseudonyms and PII. The second is the reversible pseudonymisation scheme, which allows the patient to be re-identified through the use of cryptographic mechanisms applied to the pseudonyms. The latter does not require a mapping database. There are a number of e-Health information management instances where pseudonymisation has been applied to address the challenges of permitting secondary usage of information while ensuring patient privacy and confidentiality. Here we outline some key applications of pseudonymisation in emerging domains for e-Health.

Henrici *(Henrici et al., 2006)* proposed a pseudonymisation infrastructure in which they used one-way hash functions in addressing the demands of resource scarce tags. Their approach is better than approaches based on public key cryptography.

Clinical E-science Framework (CLEF) is an E-Science programme that aims to support integrated clinical and bioscience research *(Kalra et al., 2005).* CLEF applied pseudonymisation to a repository of histories of cancer patients so that the repository can be accessed for secondary use by researchers. The pseudonymisation was used in CLEF to preserve patients's privacy and confidentiality while delivering a repository of medically rich cancer information for the purposes of scientific research.

For research purposes, especially clinical trials, patient is usually monitored during a long period of time. The disease progression and the diagnostic evolution represent extremely valuable information for researchers in clinical trials. Noumeir *(Noumeir et al., 2007)* set the objective of building a research database from de-identified clinical data while enabling the data set to be easily incremented by importing new pseudonymous data, acquired over a long period of time. They sought, through pseudonymisation, to enable the implementation of an imaging research database that can be incremented in time and propose a pseudonymisation scheme that closely follows Digital Imaging and Communication in Medicine (DICOM) standard recommendations. Noumir et al proposed the secondary usage of a radiology image electronic health record (EHR), while maintaining patient confidentiality using pseudonymisation. Malin and Sweeney *(Malin and Sweeney, 2004)* state that anonymisation and pseudonymisation lack formal proofs and expose the erosion of privacy when genomic data, either pseudonymous or anonymous, are released into a distributed e-Health environment. In their study, Malin and Sweeney applied several algorithms, which they collectively named Re-Identification of Data In Trails (REIDIT).

The REIDIT algorithms linked genomic data to named individuals in publicly available records by leveraging unique features in patient-location visit patterns. Malin and Sweeney developed algorithmic proofs of re-identification and demonstrated the susceptibility to re-identification using real world data, which is used for testing privacy protection capabilities. Their work clearly illustrates further challenges, for anonymisation and pseudonymisation, which are important elements in data analysis, data mining and knowledge discovery techniques.

CHAPTER FOUR

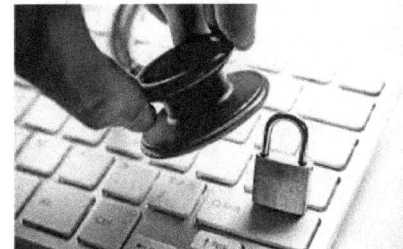

Providing Security in

Health Information Management Systems

It is believed that the Hippocratic Oath appeared in the 4th century B.C. Although there is no historical certainty about its author, it is often attributed to Hippocrates or one of its students. It has since been rewritten, to suit the values of cultures influenced by Greek medicine. It mainly exposes the broad ethical standards that a sworn physician shall uphold, and, although not mandatory, it is still traditionally used by many medical schools. From the many ethical obligations in the document, from which *"(...) I will do no harm (...)"* is probably the best known, stands the oath for secrecy:

"Whatever I see or hear in the lives of my patients, whether in connection with my professional practice or not, which ought not to be spoken of outside, I will keep secret, as considering all such things to be private."

Most professional associations and general guidelines devote great importance to doctor-patient confidentiality. This is truly important for the sake of effectiveness in that relation, as well as the safeguard of patients own rights, both ethical and legal. Doctors have earned that trust over the centuries, but in the current emergent paradigm of medical data – the transition to Information Systems, some problems are posed, namely:

• The doctor is required to write down/type the relevant information in a file whichhe does not fully control

• It no longer depends on one person to keep Information safe

O There are other professionals which may have access to the information(nurses, health technicians, clerks, orderlies, IT personnel)

O There is the problem of intrinsic HIS security

• The potential for harm from security breaches increases with the easy transport of data and simultaneous access to multiple records from one sourceSecurity and protection of patient health data, besides being demanded by patients themselves, is, in most developed countries, also required by law. In the United States, the Health Insurance Portability and Accountability Act (HIPAA) emphasizes, since 1996, the privacy of health information, and the need for its confidentiality, integrity and availability. The European Union has also issued guidelines on patient data protection, and Portugal protects health information as an individual's property, subject to confidentiality.

Handling health information is a great responsibility, and a very delicate process. HIS must be able to deal with thousands of individual records, and protect them from misuse. This is of utmost importance, since patient health data is among the most sensitive of all personal data.The effects of aggregating data into large databases are that what could be easily seen by a dozen people about one hundred people (in a small office) may be seen by one hundred people about one million (in a region). Opportunity for wrong doing increases the more people are involved. Some examples of misuse of large databases have been known for many years. Some examples are presented here:

• As banks evolve in IT structure, almost any teller in any dependency has access to account information on any bank client. Therefore it is easier to find someone interest in accepting a bribe to look for specific clients information. This may be applicable to healthcare.

• The misuse of health data can be disastrous, such as the example of a banker with a state health commission who had access to all state patients with cancer, calling its clients loans.

• Prescription systems allow for identification of trends in individuals, which may then be used to direct specific unsolicited products or services. As all patients are identifiable when they fill a prescription, the resultant database could endanger those people privacy.

• Companies holding large databases, while keeping the data private, may be bought by larger companies with interest in those databases, such as a drug company buying a health systems company.

• Many companies in the USA use medical records in their hiring decisions.

Besides security threats concerning the data privacy, HIS brings other problems on integrity and availability of data, such as hardware/software bugs, systems failure and communication problems (messages unavailable or misinterpreted).

In 2004, the Portuguese National Committee on Data protection (Comissão Nacional deProtecção de Dados - CNPD) audited 38 hospitals on personal data processing and protection. Among other problems, they found fourteen applications without password, passwords visible on stickers next to workstations on two hospitals, as well as several users stating that the passwords were, literally, their own name. This highly negative state of affairs was no surprise, as previous works on the subject had already been raising similar concerns for the last 30 years.

Generally, studies concerning the security of EHR have shown inadequate practices, urgently requiring improvement.The intrinsic value of the internet, with its promising information ubiquity, along with the possibility free and practical data communication between distinct institutions, is also its main danger, lest that information should fall into the wrong hands. Using the internet for cross-institutional communication also dramatically increases the danger of sensitive patient health information being manipulated or abused, by falling into the wrong hands. As defined by the European Union (EU):

• Data protection aims to protect the fundamental rights and freedoms of natural persons and in particular their right to privacy with respect to the processing of personal data.

• Data security aims to protect personal data against accidental or unlawful destruction or accidental loss, alteration, unauthorized disclosure or access, in particular where the processing involves the transmission of data over a network, and against all other unlawful forms of processing. This is traditionally tackled by upholding three main security characteristics[19]:

• **Confidentiality**: assurance that patient data is not made available or disclosed to unauthorized individuals. This is a serious matter, as the aggregation of information brings about new threats, with the easier access: the likelihood that information will be improperly disclosed depends on two things: its value, and the number of people who have access to it.

• **Integrity**: ensures that patient data cannot be changed or deleted by unauthorized individuals or parties. Software bugs or hardware failures can also cause data loss or wrong data.

• **Availability**: upon demand patient data can always be accessed and used by authorized people.In HIS it is also very important to be able to guarantee:

• **Authentication**: the corroboration that a person is the one claimed.

• **Non repudiation**: Someone cannot reasonably deny certain actions.

- **Accountability**: the actions of a person, especially the modifications that he/she performs on data stored in an EPR, can be traced.

The EU commission also issued the Community framework for electronic signatures, which regulates secure data exchange, and created a foundation for the legal equivalence of electronically signed documents and its hand-signed counterparts, although only through theuse of qualified and accredited electronic signatures, which guarantee such equivalence.To understand how we can start to integrate and implement all these security conceptsand properties into a HIS one must first explore what the science of Cryptography has to offerin terms of secure algorithms and communication protocols.

Cryptography

When we post a written letter, we will probably use a sealed envelope, which has the primary purpose of keeping its contents hidden to prying eyes. We generally consider the contents of personal correspondence to be private, and that the practice of sealing the envelope effectively protects its contents, even if they are not sensitive. Nowadays, it is certainly more private to use the regular mail than email, because the email systems do not protect the contents of the messages, and while they travel through multiple servers and nodes throughout the internet, until they reaches their destiny. Email can be screened and copied at any of these locations, and messages are also kept in servers, where they can be read by anyone with access to the storage. It is, however, possible to secure email, e.g. by securing the message while in transit or protecting its contents.

Both approaches generally make heavy use of cryptographic algorithms. Cryptography is a science with high historical influence for the past 2000 years. It has been used by lovers, the government and the military, with the main purpose of withholding information from unintended recipients. From a science known and practiced by few, it grew to becoming a well established academic discipline, and pervasive in modern digital societies. Contrary to items stored in a vault, encrypted messages are visible, but have their meaning hidden and therefore of no use to the eavesdroppers unless he is in possession of the means to decrypt it. Anyone may see the message, although only people in possession of the cipher key may read it, and consists of "disguising" an intelligible message in a code, by applying a set of rules and an encryption key (encryption algorithm),with no use for any person without the means to revert the process (possession of the decryption key and decryption algorithm or process).

Encrypting and decrypting a message

To make effective use of cryptography one must be aware that:

• As the keys must remain secret, there's the issue of securely distributing the keys to the intended people (senders and recipients). A key compromise will thwart security: communicating the key by an unsecure channel (email, telephone, etc.), storing the key in an accessible location (computer, post-it, etc). This means the key must be well guarded. It is pointless to secure a valuable message with a strong algorithm if the key can be easily discovered or otherwise obtained. Keys based on own names, known dates, sequences of numbers ("1234") and other common keys and passwords("password"; "password1", etc) are widely used and are automatically employed by many hacking tools.

• The Encryption Algorithm, or Cipher, as well as the keys, must be of adequate security and strength, that is, the algorithm/key must reasonably withstand expected attacks.

Steganography, or the science that studies dissimulation of messages, aids to further protect a given message, by effectively dissimulating an important and confidential encrypted message in a non sensitive, easily readable and inoffensive text or image. This adds another layer of security, comparable to having a strong vault disguised in a plain looking wall: even if a specialized burglar could know how to open it, he would have to discover its existence and location. Most of the methods used to guarantee the data security and data protection of patient health data are based on cryptographic procedures. By encoding messages written in plain text, which everyone could read, in a cipher text, which can then only be read by authorized persons, information can be securely transferred. The algorithm, which uses a person-specific parameter, the key, describes the way encryption is performed. There are a wide number of algorithms, classical and contemporaneous, that can be used to encrypt messages. They vary from the naive Caesar's substitution cipher to mathematically challenging processes, such as those used by RSA algorithms. Only some, with special interest to HIS security will be presented. There are mainly two types of encryption, symmetric and asymmetric. This is a fundamental distinction based on the keys used to encrypt and decrypt the cipher text (or cryptogram).

Symmetric cryptography

Symmetric cryptography has the advantage of being quite easy to implement and very quick to encode or decode. The same key is used in both processes. This is the classic cipher. Symmetric encryption has the disadvantage of distribution of keys, since this cannot be done over an unsecure connection. Secure key exchange is difficult, because the creation of a secure communication channel to transmit a key would depend itself on another key, so that the transmission of the keys has to be made in advance, over other channels (e.g.secure courier). There is cost and delay associated with this paradigm.

CHAPTER FIVE

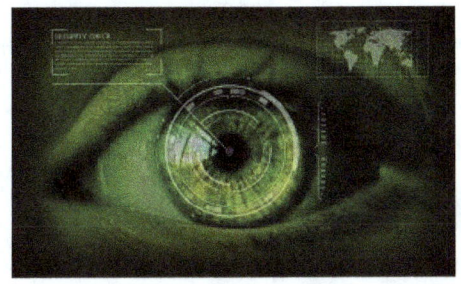

Biometrics

These are many times referred to as the "almost perfect" solution for identification, and used many times for local authentication. The key argument is that there are built around unique, unrepeatable characteristics of the human body or behavior, which can make identification of a human irrefutable. Being based in something we are, they are irrevocable, and it is very hard to erase or lose a characteristic used in biometric identification (such as removing fingerprints from fingertips). There are however various arguments against biometric technologies: They are fairly expensive to deploy; the user can not change a compromised biometric; there are various known attacks on biometric systems; there are concerns on privacy and usable biometrics also have errors, especially in identification mode when confronted with very large user databases. Another aspect, often depicted in fiction work, is the security of the owner of the biometric, as perpetrators, unable to learn or steal the feature, may physically harm the user. An example is the finger mutilation of a car owner with a fingerprint security system by car thieves in Malaysia.

Some people are unable to use biometric systems, as the enrolment success is close to, but not 100%. Examples are:

• Hand/palm recognition and fingerprints: people with no fingers, paralytic, with serious skin diseases (with no fingerprints or unreadable ones), or other diseases that impair the use of hands, such as arthritis.

• Voice recognition: some people cannot talk

• Iris or retina: there are diseases that affect this biometric and some people do not have eyes

• Face recognition: cultural hiding of women faces.Biometric technologies rely on enrollment on a system, by "capture" of certain physical or behavior characteristics (biometrics). This can be made by video, photo or other method,which, after processing, produces a template for posterior comparison.

As there are no known ways to effectively reproduce all the variables involved in collection and posterior presentation of such biometrics (position of finger or eye; subtle voice changes; lighting conditions; different equipment, etc), some tolerance shall be given, and a threshold for positive identification is created, otherwise the user has to repeat the process.

Biometric systems can identify a person by reading the biometric and comparing it to a database (1-N: identification) or to a single record (1-1: verification, e.g. after a login), different thresholds are needed, in order to reduce the number of tries needed to correct identification (false negatives or False Reject Rate - FRR), while keeping low false positives, i.e. people that successfully login identified as someone else (false Accept Rate – FAR). In identification mode the resemblance (threshold)between the trait collected and the template must be highest, or else the FAR will be unacceptable (the chance some of one's characteristics are present in another individuals template are greater the larger the database).

As a result of this, the FRR will be higher (as more resemblance is required to the stored template) and the individuals will have to repeat presentation of the trait more often.It is also possible to spoof some of the biometric systems available, by reproducing the feature of a legitimate user, which may be unaware. The main problem with this kind of attack is that we cannot hide most of the biometrics in use, as we cannot easily hide who we are.Biometric features are effectively chosen because of their ease to use, hence, to present.

Examples are successful reproduction of fingerprints left in glass or fooling facial recognition with a photo.

Token authentication

This method is based on the possession of something physical that can be uniquely associated with a certain entity and very hard to reproduce. It is very common to use smart cards as security. They are very flexible and secure: but also have some draw back. If lost, there is the possibility of system compromise. They can be, however, revoked, and re-issued. One also needs to carry it, it is not free and requires some effort to deploy and manage. If combined with a password or PIN, a token can safely store or generate multiple passwords and secret codes, which obviate the task of remembering multiple, changing passwords to one of remembering only the single password needed to access and activate the token. It also provides compromise detection, since its absence is observable (opposed to a password), and it provides added protection against denial-of-service (DoS) attacks (a person can try to login and lock multiple accounts in a login/password authentication scheme, but with the requirement of a security token, only someone with a valid active token can try to logon into the system).

Protecting HIS

We have already seen why these systems must be protected, what to have in mind when doing so and some of the technologies at our disposal.

In this section we will discuss specific problems, as well as how to deal with HIS security in its most important aspects.

Steps for a Secure HIS

Dr. Ross Anderson, in a paper for the British Medical Association policy on Security of Clinical Information Systems, regarding the introduction of a nationwide NHS (National Health Service) network, presented several principles to achieve the desirable privacy, which we discuss:

1. "Each identifiable clinical record shall be marked with an access control list naming the people or groups of people who may read it and append data to it. The system shall prevent anyone not on the access control list from accessing the record in any way."

• This principle relates to Who can access and What can they do with the data. As the databases become more ubiquitous, grows the necessity for enforcing restricted access. While 20 people in a ward may access 30 records on paper, potentially thousands of people might be able to access millions of records nationwide in an EHR without proper restrictions.

• Records could remain as they are in paper, i.e., accessible to a group of people that created the information, such as a GP (General Practitioner) and be externally accessed only by explicit consent by the patient, with or without restrictions.

• This policy must be known by the patient, so that he can make decisions regarding it.

2. " A clinician may open a record with herself and the patient on the access control list. Where a patient has been referred, she may open a record with herself, the patient and the referring clinician(s) on the access control list."

• When the patient is referred for a specific disease by his GP, there is obvious interest in that both clinicians and the patient can access the data, so the new record may have those permissions.

3. "One of the clinicians on the access control list must be marked as being responsible. Only she may alter the access control list, and she may only add other health care professionals to it."

• Other than the patient, only health care professionals may be able to access the

EHR. There must be a responsible doctor for that document, who may be the patients GP or the hospital consultant that is in charge of treating him

• Health care professionals must be both responsible and liable for misuse, and the professional status has to be defined, as some professions may not be clearly classified, such as social workers.

• When a record is transmitted and/or given access, care must be taken to ensure responsibility and liability on the receiver.

4. "The responsible clinician must notify the patient of the names on his record's access control list when it is opened, of all subsequent additions, and whenever responsibility is transferred. His consent must also be obtained,

except in emergency or in the case of statutory exemptions."

• The need for a patient to give explicit consent on the people that may access his record is difficultly overstated. In emergent situation, justification for the action has to be produced

• The responsible for the professional and/or the EHR and the patient could be notified in case of exceptional access and new additions to his "allowed" list.

5. "No-one shall have the ability to delete clinical information until the appropriate time period has expired."

• Besides setting legal mandatory persistence of records, this principle implies that records can be deleted, and sometimes, should, as in the case of a copy or access issued for the purpose of a single specialist consult.

• For some information, this could mean the lifetime of the patient (surgery report),whilst for other, this could mean a few years or less (normal blood workup).

6. "All accesses to clinical records shall be marked on the record with the subject's name, as well as the date and time. An audit trail must also be kept of all deletions."

• This feature is important in many levels. It allows for tracing and punishing of misuse,fraud or unauthorized access. It may also allow (depending on implementation) for reconstruction of some deleted data.

• The HIS must be engineered with the same care and to the same standards that are expected in life support systems, as life/death decisions can equally be made from the information conveyed from it, such as a "Do not resuscitate" notice.

7. "Information derived from record A may be appended to record B if and only if B's access control list is contained in A's."

• When a patient has two records, different information can be viewed by different people. The purpose is to keep information considered sensitive. The flagging of such hidden information (explicitly, or conspicuous lack of record parts) is controversial, as the mere knowledge of its existence could lead to inference about it. France's EHR(Dossier Medical Personnel) is dealing with such controversies.

• The release of hidden information should be considered a special action, and logged as such.

• The system should be able to prevent accidental leakage of data (such as accidentally appending clinical records to a mailing list).

8. "There shall be effective measures to prevent the aggregation of personal health information. In particular, patients must receive special notification if any person whom it is proposed to add to their access control list already has access to personal health information on a large number of people."

• This aggregation control is of utmost importance, as even in a local level, some hospitals have records in over a million people, with all users having access to that data, with less than optimal control of the access use or misuse.

• This kind of access control (or lack of it) should preclude participation in even larger networks, as "having 2,000 staff accessing a million records is bad enough; but the prospect of 200 such hospitals connected together, giving 400,000 staff access to the hospital records of most of the population, is unacceptable.".

• We should keep in mind that making data anonymous is quite hard, especially if a complete medical record is at hand, as certain medical details crossed could easily result in the identification of a single person: Caucasian, married, two daughters, 35years old, leg surgery from car accident in 2004..

• Special techniques to prevent inference from the data (statistical security) have been used in census databases, and can also be used for the purpose of mere statistical analysis.

9. "Computer systems that handle personal health information shall have a subsystem that enforces the above principles in an effective way. Its effectiveness shall be subject to evaluation by independent experts."

• All the hardware and software used in a HIS must obey all the principles above, and even enforce them. Testing for software bugs or planning for hardware failures is part of it.

• User authentication and access control is of paramount importance, as well as communications security. These features have to be tested by independent parties. This list is not an exhaustive one, yet it uncovers several key aspects that are often forgotten. We will now tackle some of the solutions to these problems.

CHAPTER SIX

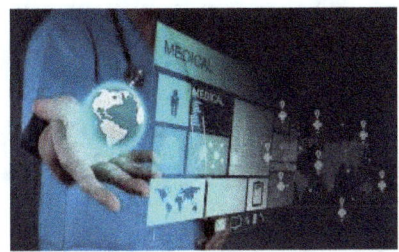

Electronic Health Records

The power of information

Health records (or clinical records) definition can be as broad as the purposes it serves: "to recall observations , to inform others, to instruct students, to gain knowledge, to monitor performance, and to justify interventions".

The Importance of Electronic Health Records

The importance of medical records is best illustrated by the way it can be put into use:

• To recall observations

O Recalling past observations or conditions is very important as a clinician has multiple patients. Apparently unassociated conditions or current medications may be of great importance when prescribing, etc.

• To inform others

O As the process of diagnosis is complicated, and the quality of information at hand influences the quality of conclusions (be it written, told by the patient,etc), information passed by a colleague with training aids in the speed of treatment. The clinician can make deduction and reason on the basis of previous findings, instead of having to repeat the steps necessary to reach a correct diagnosis.

• To instruct students

O Medical knowledge is very vast. One of the ways medical students learn is by studying and discussing clinical cases, which makes it easier to develop clinical skills and to incorporate knowledge.

• To gain knowledge

O Progress in health care would not be possible without clinical studies, and the analysis of its findings. Medical knowledge began by basic observations on conditions and patients and evolved to complex clinical trials, in which control and manipulation of variables permits precise and accurate conclusions.

•To monitor performance

O The performance of a drug, a health care institution, a diagnostic test, etc., maybe ascertained from the proper records of patients, from which we may try to extrapolate conclusions, given a correct methodology.

•To justify interventions

O Medical history can be used to justify, for instance, the use of a drug in light of a personal condition that precludes the use of others, or a more aggressive treatment plan when conservative ones failed, etc.

Electronic Health Records (EHR), computerized records, electronic charts, etc. refer to a medical record on digital format. Electronic records may be as simple as a scanned bitmap image of the actual paper record, or as advanced as a fully interactive, searchable file, with multiple data input yields (images, reports, free writing, selectable items, etc). To most people, information concerning its health is stored on the providers, scattered in all visited institutions, thus making it very difficult to have instantaneous access to all data and creating "information islands". The paradigm of health records on paper makes it even harder to access and distribute all information related to a given patient. Furthermore, the amount of data generated nowadays overwhelms traditional storage, especially because of imaging studies [98], not only in a physical way, but because of the growing difficulty in retrieving specific data in timely fashion.

The Ideal situation would be to have a secure, ubiquitous, complete, reliable and interoperable medical record. This is very difficult to procure. Security is an mandatory issue,especially if ubiquity is a reality. The fact that a patient private, law protected, medical history can be accessed from everywhere in the internet makes the framework used for service implementation critical in terms of security and requiring services planning and testing,because there is a need to protect The EHR confidentiality and integrity, while making it available to the right people.

The EHR has been a key research field in medicine and medical informatics for many years. A commonly used definition is that EHR is "digitally stored healthcare information about an individual's lifetime with the purpose of supporting continuity of care, education and research, and ensuring confidentiality at all times". EHRs are repositories of electronically maintained information about individuals' lifetime health status and healthcare, stored so they can serve the multiple legitimate users of the record. These are rather idealistic concepts. Meeting them requires interoperable solutions that integrate and connect partial EHRs and clinical information stored by various healthcare providers and other actors. Current, operational EHRs include information such as observations, laboratory tests, diagnostic imaging reports, treatments, therapies, drugs prescribed, dispensed and administered, patient identifying information and demographics, legal permissions, allergies and the identities of healthcare professionals and provider organisations who have provided healthcare. This information is stored in various electronic formats using a multitude of medical information systems available on the market.

Given the complexity of the comprehensive definitions and features of EHRs, we prefer to talk about EHR systems rather than unique, stand-alone complete EHRs. **An EHR system can include parts of a comprehensive record, allow limited or extensive sharing of information, or be part of a particular healthcare provider organisation. It is seldom all the health-related data about people, often envisaged by grand strategies.** Although partial, such EHRs are substantial and successful where they are currently in routine operation. Experience gathered from these current solutions is indispensable in identifying the real benefits from EHRs and in clarifying future requirements and potential. In the report, the terms 'EHR' and 'EHR system' are used interchangeably.

E-Prescribing

Like the term EHR, e-Prescribing is not a well-defined fixed term, but extends over a wide variety of solutions, often related to individual activities such as prescribing, dispensing, and advice on controlled drugs. The EHR IMPACT study takes a broad perspective of e-Prescribing. It sees it as part of a wider health information system, potentially based on EHRs, and includes prescribing policies, clinical decisions, decision support, dispensing, advice to patients and careers, and the processes and roles of each stakeholder needed to convert prescribing decisions into administered medications. These extend across primary care and hospital settings, and are interoperable with the equivalent EHRs.

Definitions of e-Prescribing

E-Health Initiative defined electronic prescribing as "the use of computing devices to enter, modify, review, and output or communicate drug prescriptions". The Initiative distinguishes six levels of e-Prescribing, each expanding on the functionalities of the previous one.

The distinct feature of the definition is the focus on medications. The definition explicitly states that e-Prescribing is about drug prescriptions. In the UK, Connecting for Health (CfH) also defines e-Prescribing with a focus on medications only, but includes more than the prescribing process alone. At the same time, e-Prescribing includes "aiding the choice of medicines *and other therapies*", moving the concept away from the strict focus on medications.

E-Prescribing and Computerized Physician Order Entry (CPOE)

E-Prescribing solutions fit with CPOE initiatives. These set medication regimes alongside all other treatments and diagnostic activities. CPOE is **a process where the instructions of physicians regarding the treatment of patients under their care are entered electronically and communicated**

directly to responsible individuals or services. Before CPOE, such orders were hand-written or orally communicated, sometimes leading to medical errors. CPOE can be implemented as part of a larger hospital information system (HIS) or clinical information system (CIS) and thus be interoperable with EHRs, medical records and other patient information. A common feature is that ePrescribing and CPOE are part of EHR systems.

The concept of interoperable EHR and e-Prescribing systems

Translating the previous concepts and definitions into operational use by the study, needed pragmatic definitions of EHR and e-Prescribing interoperability levels:

1) **Potential interoperability** involves EHR and/or e-Prescribing solutions and use of technology standards allowing information to be shared, but without actual exchange taking place

2) **Limited connectivity** refers to a situation in which not all features and levels of interoperability, as defined above, are achieved, yet some information exchange and sharing is practiced

3) **Extended actual connectivity** comes close to real interoperation by using interoperability to exchange and share information and knowledge with other actors in the health system.

This facilitates collaboration and change in clinical and working practices and roles, as well as creating and expanding multi-disciplinary teams.

Privacy, Security, And Electronic Health Records

Your health care provider may be moving from paper records to electronic health records (EHRs) or may be using EHRs already. EHRs allow providers to use information more effectively to improve the quality and efficiency of your care, but EHRs will not change the privacy protections or security safeguards that apply to your health information.

EHRs and Health Information

EHRs are electronic versions of the paper charts in your doctor's or other health care provider's office. An EHR may include your medical history, notes, and other information about your health including your symptoms, diagnoses, medications, lab results, vital signs, immunizations, and reports from diagnostic tests such as x-rays.

Providers are working with other doctors, hospitals, and health plans to find ways to share that information. The information in EHRs can be shared with other organizations involved in your care if the computer systems are set up to talk to each other. Information in these records should only be shared for purposes authorized by law or by you.

You have privacy rights whether your information is stored as a paper record or stored in an electronic form. The same federal laws that already protect your health information also apply to information in EHRs.

Benefits of EHRs

Whether your health care provider is just beginning to switch from paper records to EHRs or is already using EHRs within the office, you will likely experience one or more of the following benefits:

> ➤ **Improved Quality of Care.** As your doctors begin to use EHRs and set up

ways to securely share your health information with other providers, it will make it easier for everyone to work together to make sure you are getting the care you need. For example:

- Information about your medications will be available in EHRs so that health care providers don't give you another medicine that might be harmful to you.

- EHR systems are backed up like most computer systems, so if you are in an area affected by a disaster, like a hurricane, your health information can be retrieved.

- EHRs can be available in an emergency. If you are in an accident and are unable to explain your health history, a hospital that has a system may be able to talk to your doctor's system. The hospital will get information about your medications, health issues, and tests, so decisions about your emergency care are faster and more informed.

➤ **More Efficient Care.** Doctors using EHRs may find it easier or faster to track your lab results and share progress with you. If your doctors' systems can share information, one doctor can see test results from another doctor, so the test doesn't always have to be repeated. Especially with x-rays and certain lab tests, this means you are at less risk from radiation and other side effects. When tests are not repeated unnecessarily, it also means you pay less for your health care in co-payments and deductibles.

➢ **More Convenient Care.** EHRs can alert providers to contact you when it is time for certain screening tests. When doctors, pharmacies, labs, and other members of your health care team are able to share information, you may no longer have to fill out all the same forms over and over again, wait for paper records to be passed from one doctor to the other, or carry those records yourself.

Ensuring Your Electronic Health Information Secure

Most of us feel that our health information is private and should be protected. The federal government put in place the Health Insurance Portability and Accountability Act of 1996 (HIPAA) Privacy Rule to ensure you have rights over your own health information, no matter what form it is in. The government also created the HIPAA Security Rule to require specific protections to safeguard your electronic health information. A few possible measures that can be built in to EHR systems may include:

- "Access control" tools like passwords and PIN numbers, to help limit access to your information to authorized individuals.

- "Encrypting" your stored information. That means your health information cannot be read or understood except by those using a system that can "decrypt" it with a "key."

- An "audit trail" feature, which records who accessed your information, what changes were made and when.

Finally, federal law requires doctors, hospitals, and other health care providers to notify of a "breach." The law also requires the health care provider to notify the Secretary of Health and Human Services. If a breach affects more than 500 residents of a state or jurisdiction, the health care provider must also notify prominent media outlets serving the state or jurisdiction. This requirement helps patients know if something has gone wrong with the protection of their information and helps keep providers accountable for EHR protection.

CHAPTER SEVEN

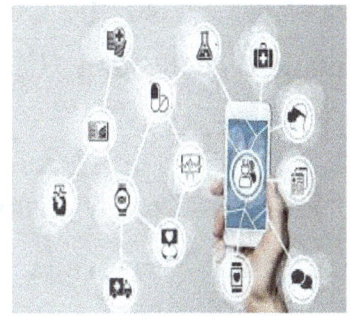

Mobile Health (mHealth)

Medical and public health practice supported by mobile devices, such as mobile phones, patient monitoring devices, personal digital assistants (PDAs), and otherwireless devices. mHealth stands for mobile-based solutions that deliver health. Mobile health (mHealth) is an essential element of electronic health (eHealth)

mHealth is important because it makes healthcare practices accessible to the public through mobile communication technologies in a variety of ways (e.g., providing healthcare information, collecting health data, observing patients, etc.

mHealth aims to improve care by making health information easily accessible for patients with long-term conditions (chronic disease) such as diabetes. There are currently more than 165,000 mobile health apps publicly available in major app stores. The vast majority of which are designed for patients.The top 2 categories are wellness management and disease management apps. other categories include: self diagnosis, medication reminder, and electronic patient portal apps.

Mobile Health, or mHealth, describes the use of mobile and wireless communication technologies to improve healthcare delivery, outcomes, and research. 259,000 mHealth apps are available on app stores. 3.2 billion downloads annually.

❖ **Success Factors in mhealth:**

- aim
- user
- location
- regulations and content
- platform
- Idea
- marketing and support of application

❖ **Barriers and issues: (5-7)**

- regulatory

- Privacy and Security

- Integration

- Reliability

- Accessibility

- Acceptability

- Usability

- Confidentiality

- Integrity

- Knowledge Sharing

- Systems Flexibility

- lack of teamwork

- poor security

- high price

- Lack of clinician involvement

- poor attention to usability

❖ m-Health services architectures

Typical m-Health services architectures (presented in Fig. 1) use the Internet and Web services to provide interaction among doctors and patients.

A physician or a patient can easily access the same medical record anytime and anywhere through his/her personal computer, tablet, or smartphone.

The patient can contact the physician in case of an emergency, or even, have access to medical registers or appointments regardless of time and place.

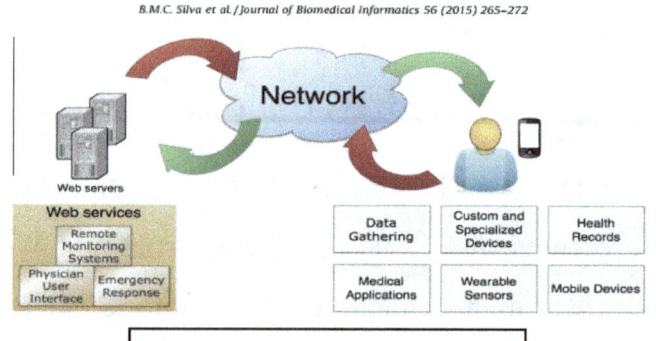

B.M.C. Silva et al./Journal of Biomedical Informatics 56 (2015) 265–272

Methodological Review Mobile-health: A review of current state in 2015

mHealth Goals:

- Develop patient-centered healthcare delivery

- Increased self-management of illness

- Reduced number of hospital beds occupied

- Remote monitoring and smart diagnosis

- Improved disease management

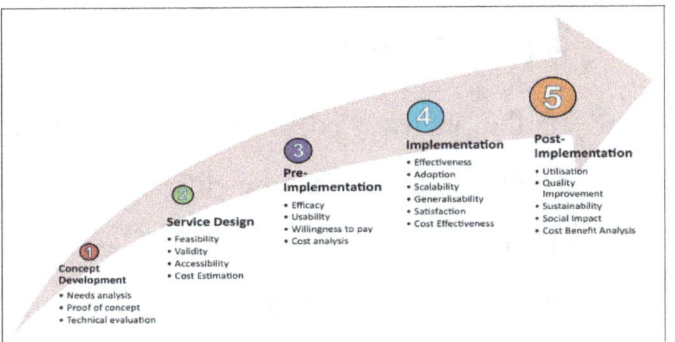

❖ suggesting a technology-based solution for a health or medical problem (Stage 1: Concept development).

❖ how the service delivery model should be modified/re-designed to accommodate the proposed intervention (Stage 2: Service design).

❖ the efficacy of the proposed model of care/service should be studied under a controlled environment (Stage 3: Pre implementation).

❖ If the efficacy of the intervention is established, it can be the subject of subsequent study in real-world settings in which the intervention is implemented and its effectiveness is studied (Stage 4: Implementation).

❖ After implementation of a telehealth intervention, several research approaches can be taken to examine the impact and sustainability of the system (Stage 5: Post-implementation).

Diabetes:

❖ The majority of mHealth disease management interventions have focused on diabetes.Patients living with diabetes experience difficulties associated with poor knowledge about their condition and the need to maintain a strict lifestyle.Diabetes, as a disease, is associated with many complications; therefore, education, management, and control of diabetes is of vital importance.

mHealth could help diabetic patients make decisions necessary for optimal insulin dosing and promote self-management. self-management aims to involve patients in their long-term care

Mobile Application (App)

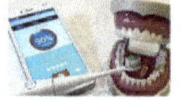

Kolibree toothbrush: Record every brush stroke. Sends your dental report to your smartphone via Bluetooth

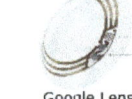

Google Lenses: Contact Detects glucose in tears

Smartphone-based ultrasound imaging

Withings Aura: Built for people suffering from insomnia. Tracks body movements, Breathing motion, noice pollution & room temperature

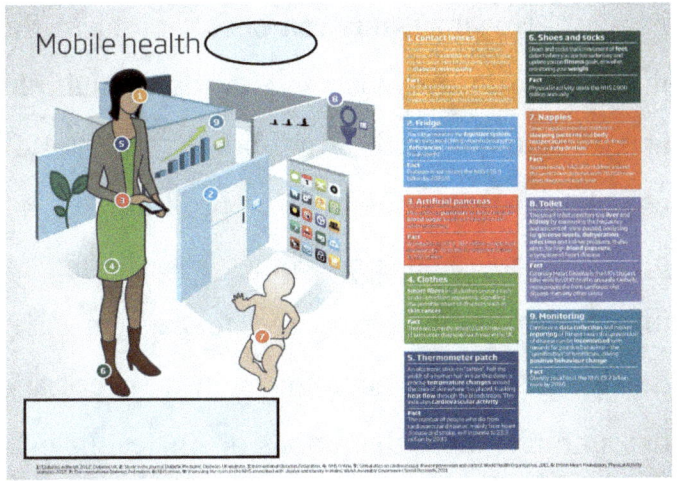

Continuum of mHealth tools

Continuum of mHealth tools

Although many mHealth apps currently exist, there is still a need for improvements. The utilisation of mHealth tools continues to increase. However, this can pose a problem for those who do not wish to download multiple apps. There is a need for uniformity and ease of use for patients. With the proliferation of mHealth tools and apps comes a scattering of information, which may lead to gaps in care. Lastly, a comprehensive tool will be necessary to simplify the integration of mHealth into standard practice of care.

The pace of uptake, development and utilisation of mHealth across the globe is and will continue to be varied. The implementation of access technologies will likely continue, but diagnostics and maintenance is only one part of health care approaches to develop interventions or enact systematic change will still be necessary.

Wearables

Wearable technology can be defined as items (often with electronic capabilities) worn with acceptable function and aesthetic properties, consisting of a simple interface to perform set tasks to satisfy needs of a specific group. These may be worn as an accessory, incorporated in clothing, or as an implant (more permanent and invasive).

The commercialization of wearable technologies has drastically increased during the last 5 years, as the size of computers has decreased and the development of smart sensors has enabled the creation of small and precise trackers for a wide array of functions ranging from smart glasses to smart bracelets. At the core of this wearable technology evolution is the wearable health tech, which is becoming more and more prone to technology. Many companies have started developing wearable devices towards implementing more sufficient ways of providing healthcare. The various range of wearable devices are being developed in order to fill a void where human error is present. In this thesis the focus will be in explaining what wearable technology really includes, as well as both the future prospects and problems for wearable technology in healthcare. As this technology is still in its early adaption phase, various kinds of information are needed about the subject to change people's perceptions about wearable technology acceptance in healthcare.

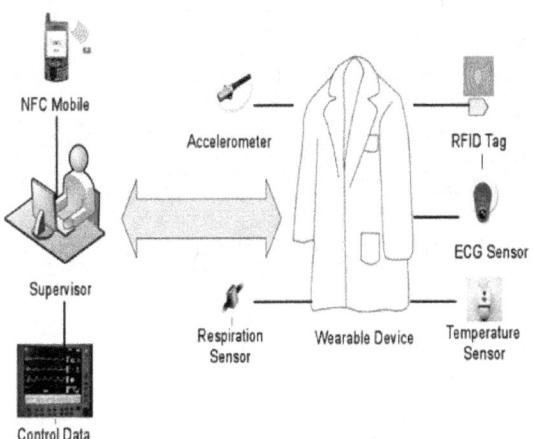

Characteristics of a wearable device

Consumer wearable technology has a strong focus on health and fitness. The increased availability and ability to monitor physiological signals allow us to gain closer insights in our health. It also enables the use of new intervention techniques to influence our behaviour. Even smartwatches like the new Apple Watch, whose main purpose is not fitness tracking, are equipped with biosensors to monitor heart rate and steps made over the day. This reflects the strong interest of individuals in wanting to know about their own health and fitness

Wearable Devices Wearable devices can be divided into two distinct categories: 'wearable computers' and 'smart textiles'. Wearable computers are fashion accessories that contain the necessary electronics, usually they are bracelets or watches. They enable consumers to carry out tasks in a relatively unobtrusive and socially acceptable way leading to increased levels of productivity or enjoyment. The 'smart textiles', according to Hertleer, Langenhove and Schwartz (2012), are electronics woven into the fabric, enabling products to measure and/or react to stimuli from the user or environment. The advantage that smart textiles possess over 12 smart computers is that they can be worn comfortably for longer periods of time without skin irritation even though they lose in the range of possible user interactions. Therefore, they are more appropriate for long term monitoring applications or for circumstances where aesthetics is highly important

Wearable technology components

Several elements are required for wearable technologies. Sensors, actuators and controllers (often microcontrollers), a power source, and software (data acquisition, use, transfer, and storage) are considered the main components. Each component can be tailored to a specific application based on function. Combining these components results in a single wearable device that can be worn as accessories

Wearable technology challenges and issues:

Accessibility, confidentiality, and security of highly personal information collected with wearable technology is a concern. Hacking devices for information is a potential risk and appropriate protection is necessary (e.g. anti-virus software). Potential emission/radiation from electrical-networks needs to be managed. These issues are being addressed. For example, fabric area networks produce systems restricted to the fabric surface for greater control, enhanced information security, reduced interference, and minimised radiation/emission exposure from electronic devices). However, transmitting information to an external device (e.g. phone, computer) is desirable for interpreting, collating, and storing data under some situations. 3.2 Timeline of developments Wearable technology has existed for hundreds of years at least since the 15th century. Trends include miniaturisation, increased mobilisation, and incorporation of multifunctional capabilities. Further, functionalisation of accessories already frequently worn by individuals (e.g. spectacles) is more common than 'new' accessories.

Wearable technology in Healthcare, Wellness and Fitness:

In Healthcare concept, Wearables surrounding health applications need to be accurate and reliable because data collected may be used for diagnosing, monitoring, and/or treating patients. Risks of inaccurate data providing misinformation could be life threatening. Health-related information should be preventive, personalised, patient-centred, and precise, to efficiently and effectively provide information to the wearer or medical professionals as appropriate. Wearable devices need to perform in a way similar to, or superior to traditional devices.

Wearable technology for health care presents a number of potential benefits including a convenient and less obtrusive alternative to care in clinical settings (e.g. using fibre-optic sensors in magnetic resonance imaging scanners. Post-operative care and rehabilitation in clinical settings following a debilitating event can be facilitated. For example, a bionic glove has been developed with functional electrical stimulation capabilities to assist hand rehabilitation following a spinal cord injury or stroke. Medical care can be transferred to home and other external environments with selected technology, permitting continuous monitoring and treatment administered through individual's daily life. Automation of monitoring and treatment is also possible reducing requirements of the wearer, particularly desirable for people who may be forgetful or those with especially time-constrained lives. Information collected in 'normal' settings is likely to provide better indication of an individual's condition than an atypical reading in a doctor's office. Isolated individuals, those with limited access to resources (e.g. developing countries, rural areas, military), or high demand for medical care (e.g. disease outbreaks, natural disasters) can be assisted with some form of wearable technology. Dealing with susceptibility to illness (e.g. elderly) or chronic conditions (e.g. Parkinson's disease, diabetes, deafness, and blindness) can be simplified with wearable devices. This is particularly topical with ageing populations (lower number of births, longer expected life span) resulting in a demand for independence. Mental disorders (e.g. anxiety) can be better managed with wearable devices which encourage relaxation. Thus physiological and psychological aspects of health can be improved. The health care wearables sector is expected to reach US$4.4 billion in 2019 and US$4.5 billion by 2020. Leading companies contributing to this sector include *Gentag®, Google®, Intel® (three United States based companies), Polar Electro® (Finland), Omron® (Japan), LifeWatch® (Switzerland), Philips® (Netherlands), and WithingsTM (France). TextronicsTM (United States based company)* has produced devices for individuals to assist weight loss and heart health. Companies contributing to the health sector indicate country/regional participation: the United States of America, Europe (Finland, Switzerland, Netherlands, France), and Japan. The Asia Pacific area has been reported as the fastest growing in the medical sector with a 23.8% compound annual growth rate for 2014 to 2020, but start and end estimates have not been identified.

The fitness field is one of the most familiar wearable applications that we experience every day. In practice, the majority of related products including software and applications have been launched in this field. Furthermore, there have been many attempts to converge wearable technology for expanding this market. By combining position-based tracking such as a global positioning system (GPS), motion tracking using accelerometers and gyroscopes, and physiological tracking via heart rate monitors, which are the most fundamental utilization included in wearable devices, user logs such as distance moved, calories consumed, and average speed can be calculated. Furthermore, the use of physical posture detection sensors can propose the optimum exercise routine after examining whether users are exercising correctly. Wearable technology encourages active and healthy lifestyles, so it can be utilized to monitor physical activities to improve the health and physical strength of those who need exercises such as obese people or those who lack exercise due to work; it can also facilitate clinical intervention.

Many research groups have looked into the possibility of wearables to accelerate healthcare beyond simple fitness assistive applications used by individuals. An extensive study on remote monitoring applications based on wearables has been conducted in the healthcare field, mainly for the elderly who have difficulty in their daily lives and patients with movement disorders due to fatal chronic diseases such as Parkinson's disease, stroke, or dementia. These patients need constant assistance from guardians such as family members or caregivers because they cannot live normally without help. Hence, related studies aim to improve their quality of life by monitoring their health condition, behavior, and signs of worsening symptoms, while also providing information about condition changes over time, thereby enabling independent and comfortable daily life activities. In addition, it helps with the management of chronic diseases by exchanging information about patients' health conditions in real time among patients, doctors, and family members. Wearable devices attached to patients play an important role in improving diagnosis and treatment methods by monitoring physiological data such as heart rate, blood pressure, oxygen saturation, respiration rate, body temperature, and electrical skin reaction over a long time. The parameters extracted from these measurements can provide indices for health conditions of patients with significant diagnostic value. Until comparatively lately, the constant monitoring of physiological parameters was only possible at hospitals, but patient data now can be monitored in real time during normal home life. The technological development can help doctors determine the symptoms of patients more accurately.

The wearables can now be utilized even in the remote rehabilitation treatment field. For example, intensive long-term rehabilitation is a major factor in ensuring the recovery of reduced exercise function after the onset of a stroke. Tracking the change in conditions of exercise functions can be utilized as a feedback means to guide appropriate rehabilitation processes. Furthermore, remote home-rehabilitation applications based on wearables increase the time that patients can stay Sustainability at home instead of visiting hospitals for the purpose of treatment, thereby reducing treatment costs. These remote applications can also be utilized to monitor the safety status of patients with movement disorders. A broad range of wearable devices that are integrated with wireless networks can track and analyze patients' movement status such as walking, spotting movement difficulties, thereby automatically sending alarms or urgent call messages to their family members or caregivers when patients fall or experience a sudden shock. These applications can both detect physiological states of patients and enhance their sensitivity of detection by combining with motion sensors such as accelerometer mounted in wearable sensors in the patient's home environment. They may help patients with their daily living and reduce the stress on family members by providing accurate information after analyzing data streams in order to monitor health conditions, daily living activities, and urgent situations.

For the elderly

Most elderly persons want to continue living in their own homes with the help of geriatric home care service. This sets great demands on our health care system. This is probably the biggest potential for wearable technology in the future. Using wearable technology to monitor the health of the elderly who are not staying in hospitals is where the biggest potential for improving healthcare in general lays. The elderly are being socially excluded from the newest trends such as mobile applications as the majority of the new efforts are being targeted at younger adults. Kandler et. Al. (2015) found out that elderly have very different personality types compared to younger adults, resulting in decreased openness and hesitation in willingness of adopting new technologies. This issue could be resolved by integrating smart wearable devices into their daily lives. It is a known fact that elderlies in general have difficulties in handling new technologies; technological advancements have been burgeoning during the 21th century and the senior citizens have troubles keeping up with the pace of the newest trends

Recommended validation process for wearable healthcare devices.

Step 1 – Content Validation: There needs to be a needs assessment for a particular device, which can be identified from the literature, based upon review of its functions. Expert opinion can be used to determine whether the device will be suitable for its intended use.

Step 2 – Reliability Assessment should take place with evaluation of the device features, limitations and cost effectiveness.

Step 3 – Implementation should follow after discussions with Healthcare Technology Assessment and clinical trials comparing the device to the gold standard method

CONTENT VALIDATION	RELIABILITY ASSESSMENT	IMPLEMENTATION
•Needs Assessment •Literature Review •Identification of Device •Review of Functions •Expert Opinion	•Portability •Battery Life •Data storage •Feasability of Use •Patient Compliance •Limitations •Ease of Wearability •'Clothing accessory' •Cost-effectiveness	•Discussion with Healthcare Technology Assessment •Clinical Trial comparing to current gold-standard

Validation process for wearable healthcare devices.

Wearables are a rapidly evolving product segment. Wearable technology offers much promise to improve the delivery of healthcare for both patients and care providers, especially with the advent of regulated, wearable medical devices. We are on the cusp of rapid innovation being brought about by large players that are offering standard platforms for wearable technology. This will reduce the cost of regulatory compliance and propel the industry to the more stable ground of wearables as regulated medical devices instead of merely consumer electronics devices. It is high time that regulators, developers and healthcare providers embrace the potential of these new technologies to improve the delivery of care to patients.

CHAPTER EIGHT

Public Health Opportunities in Health Information Exchange

Public health participation in health information exchanges presents opportunities for both short-term and transformative impacts on the health system.

Health Information Exchange

Health information exchange (HIE) describes both (1) the act of sharing of clinical and administrative health care data between interested stakeholders and (2) the actual health information technologies and systems that facilitate this sharing. There have been multiple iterations of this concept over the past three decades, starting with the Community Health Information Networks of the 1980s, the Regional Health Information Organizations of the late 1990s - early 2000s, and now the health information exchanges that exist in various forms and offer services ranging from basic connectivity to more advanced functions such as master patient indexes, provider directories, trust services, e-prescribing, and public health reporting. The Health Information Technology for Economic and Clinical Health (HITECH) Act of 2009 has helped to promote HIE by including HIE reporting as a Meaningful Use Stage to measure and funding the State HIE Cooperative Agreement Program which provides funding for a state designated entity (SDE) to plan and build HIE capacity. There are many challenges to address. Data and messaging standards are required for semantic interoperability. The complexity of information privacy and security policies and regulations increases proportionately with the number of HIE participants. Governance and sustainability are also major challenges that must be met. The future of HIE is promising. The increasing adoption of EHR systems creates a pool of electronic health data that can support public health needs, such as automated reporting for communicable diseases, predictive analysis for syndromic surveillance, and population health reporting.

National interest in health information exchange has arisen from the convergence of four historic trends: a demand for health care cost containment and quality improvement, the urgent desire for better surveillance and response to public health emergencies, the emergence of technologies capable of providing electronic person-centric health information on demand, and the development of the Internet and technologies that can link information between users with little regard to distance, hardware, or software platforms.

The ability to securely and rapidly exchange patient clinical information between health care providers has been demonstrated in a few model programs. Such collaborations have variously been called local health information infrastructures, regional health information exchanges, sub-network organizations, and regional health information organizations, depending on their scope. No matter what they are called, it appears today that affordable technology solutions are within our grasp, necessary standards are being established (vocabulary, data coding, message format, etc.), and communities are actively forming health information exchanges.

In one regard, the stars appear aligned; there is unprecedented interest among both the public and private sectors in the development and adoption of common architectural standards for health system interoperability.

Patients in Health Information Exchange

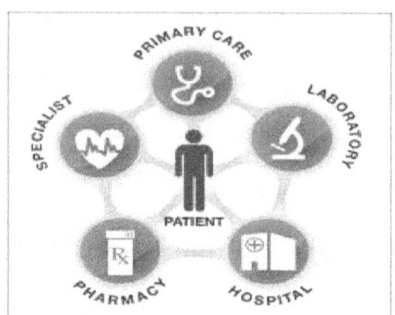

Some have argued that at this early stage, health information exchanges are essentially business-to-business (B2B) ventures. That is, they facilitate health care organizations and their providers in the task of delivering care. Consequently, involving patients directly in the flow of electronic patient information unnecessarily complicates the picture. Others have argued that patient-centered, patient-controlled applications are critical to maximizing the impact of the health information exchange on care, cost, quality, and safety.

The information in a health information exchange could potentially support personalized health promotion and disease prevention tools that are far more effective than current approaches. Thus, there may be a link between patient access to health information exchange information and public health outcomes. Since there is an inevitable trade-off between privacy and information access, patient-controlled applications may also help gain patient acceptance for exchanging their information in the first place.

Public Health in Health Information Exchange

Given the interdependence of public health agencies and health care organizations, early consideration of public health functionality of health information exchanges can help ensure that benefits to both are maximized. Public health refers both to a set of legal constructs, as well as a more general concept related to population health. The police powers and obligations of government to protect public health originate in common law and are controlled primarily by local and state statutes.

The stars appear aligned; there is unprecedented interest among both the public and private sectors in the development and adoption of common architectural standards for health system interoperability.

health functions relate to personal health information and personal care, such as required reporting of health conditions by physicians and laboratories to public health authorities, and the latter's responsibility to advise providers in the face of a community health threat.

Public health is also defined more broadly as ***"what we, as a society, do collectively to assure the conditions in which people may be healthy."*** This recognizes that protecting and promoting health is necessarily a shared responsibility. Government must inform, regulate, and coordinate overall efforts, but, in the final analysis, public health outcomes rely as much on actions of employers, schools, health care providers, business owners and individuals.

Modern terminology refers to the "public health system" in which government is but one (albeit central) player. Indeed, the work of public health agencies is increasingly characterized by providing health information and knowledge to other agencies, upon which they rely to perform important public health activities. The contemporary public health model is characterized above all else by inter-dependency. Both of these visions of public health (legal mandates and communal action) should inform the interaction of public health with health information exchanges.

Public health is described as having three core functions: assessment of health status, policy development related to health, and assurance of needed conditions and services. The public health system should provide essential services to each community:

Monitor health status to identify and solve community health problems. information resources and knowledge management; providing access to reference materials, decision-support, and distance learning; alerting and communications enabling greater collaboration among agencies and other health system partners; and response systems supporting both emergency and routine public health business processes.

Public Health and Health Information Exchange: A Two-Way Relationship

Every visual conceptualization of a health information exchange has shown at least a one-way information arrow leading from the health information exchange to public health, indicating passive data listening.

This overlooks the potential for public health to provide substantial information that is useful to clinicians at the point of service (e.g., both information related to specific patients, such as immunization records or case management information) as well as higher-level knowledge derived from population level information (e.g., illness trends or expert guidance). Public health agencies typically manage large amounts of data of great potential value to health care providers, but struggle with converting and delivering it as useful information for the practice of medicine. Standardized electronic information could radically improve the process. It would enable near-real-time data capture, partial automation of data analysis to create useful information, and rapid transmission of that information to providers. Further, knowledge could be delivered in a form and context most useful at the point of care (e.g., "This patient lacks a record of any MMR immunization"; or "Consider diagnosis of pertussis in light of patient's symptoms and current outbreak"). Additionally, public health agencies may have unique legal or organizational attributes (e.g., a trusted neutral party experienced with maintaining confidential health information; a potential connector to public sector high-bandwidth infrastructure) that could substantially aid health information exchange governance and architecture.

While public health agencies may have unique attributes that would warrant involvement in health information exchanges, many questions remain. For example, do some public health agencies have health care regulatory roles that interfere or conflict with their ability to be full partners in the health information exchange governance or information exchange? Do certain health information exchange business models or information architecture characteristics either enhance or inhibit the achievement of community- level public health applications? Is it most practical to sort public health/health information exchange functionality based on types of information to be exchanged, the types of health problems or populations to be addressed, or the types of functions (e.g., alerting, decision-support, case management) to be performed?

CHAPTER NINE

TELEMEDICINE

Definitions & concepts used in Telemedicine

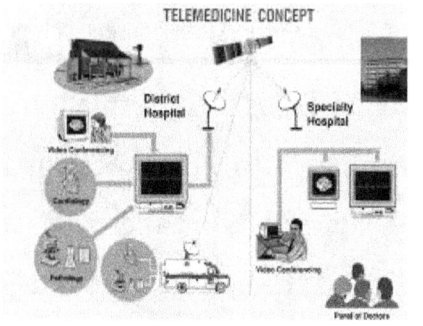

The World Health Organization defines Telemedicine as, "The delivery of healthcare services, where distance is a critical factor, by all healthcare professionals using information and communication technologies for the exchange of valid information for diagnosis, treatment and prevention of disease and injuries, research and evaluation, and for the continuing education of healthcare providers, all in the interests of advancing the health of individuals and their communities".

Tele-health

Tele-health is the use of electronic information and telecommunications technologies to support long-distance clinical health care, patient and professional health-related education and training, public health and health administration.

Tele-consultation

Tele-consultation is the use of information and communications technology to enable clinical consultation between geographically separated individuals such as health care professionals and their patients or health care professionals engaged in diagnostic, mentoring, or other clinical decision-making activities related to the delivery of health care services.

Tele-monitoring

A real time and live interactive monitoring (evaluation) of technique(s) or procedure(s) of an applicant seeking privileges, or a surgeon seeking to certify or document his competence in a specific technique or procedure(s). The Tele-monitor is in one location and the surgeon to be evaluated is in another. The Tele-monitor must have the ability to see the performance of the procedure or technique being executed by the student in real time. The Tele-monitor and the applicant must have the ability tq verbally communicate during the session.

Tele-monitoring may be used as an adjunct to proctoring in the privileging process but should not alone be a substitute for proctoring to determine competency. Integration of Tele-monitoring into the proctoring process may reduce, but not eliminate, the number of on-site proctored cases required.

Tele-monitoring assumes that the ability of the Tele-monitor to physically intervene at the site of the primary procedure is not possible without the telecommunications interface

Tele-treatment

Treatment provided to the patient through Telemedicine. The specialist at the Specialty Centre could advise the consulting doctor at the

Consulting Centre about the course of treatment to be taken.

Patient Information Record (PIR)

All information pertaining to the patient for providing care using Telemedicine. This included clinical as well as non-clinical information.

Clinical Information

This includes history of the illness, associated signs and symptoms clinical observations, clinical interventions, diagnostics and treatments etc., relevant for providing care, using Telemedicine.

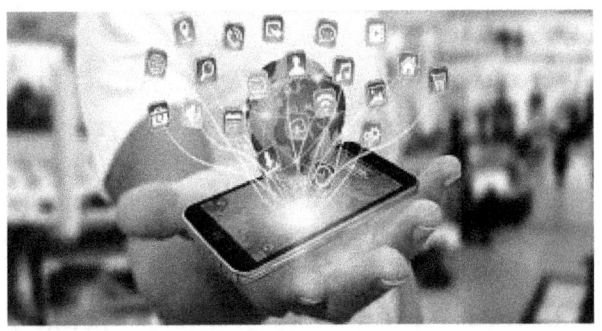

Non-clinical Information

Non-clinical information include information about the patient's environment demographic information, life style, occupation or about related people, etc., where this is relevant for providing care using Telemedicine.

Tele-medicine Consultation Centre (TCC) .

Telemedicine Consulting Centre is the site where the patient is present. In a Telemedicine Consulting Centre, equipment for scanning /

converting, transformation, communicating for medical information of the patient can be available but it is not essential. A Telemedicine Consulting Centre usually has a General Practitioner or in very remote locations a Registered Medical Practitioner who will be able to communicate to the TSC the symptoms/problems of the patient.

Telemedicine Specialty Centre (TSC)

Telemedicine Specialty Centre is a site, where the specialist is present. He can interact with the patient present in the remote site and view his reports and monitor his progress. A Specialty Centre is generally located in a Specialty or Super Specialty hospital catering for specific specialties or all specialties.

Healthcare network

Communications network designed to suit the health sector and the provision of health information via an assortment of electronic devices (computers, printers, scanners, etc.) connected for mutual exchange of digital information.

Telemedicine System

Telemedicine system consists of an interface between hardware, software and communication channel to eventually bridge two geographical locations to exchange information and enable tele-consultancy between two locations. The hardware consists of computer, printer, scanner, video conferencing equipment etc. The software enables the acquisition of patient information (images, reports, films etc.). The communication channel enables the connectivity whereby two locations can connect to each other.

Tele-diagnostics

Tele-diagnostics is the use of ~formation and communications technologies to enable the diagnosis orca patient between geographically separated individuals. Tele-diagnostics is usually a real time and live dialogue between the specialist and the doctor at the remote site with regard to the diagnosis of the patient's illness. The specialist is in one location and the consulting doctor/patient is in another. But it is also possible that Tele-diagnostics could be of a

Store and forward type where the patient's information is transmitted to the TSC and the specialist gives his expert opinion after a specific period of time. This could happen in circumstances where the specialist was not available at the time of receipt of patient information at the TSC or there was a communication breakdown and it was not possible to give the opinion in real time.

Store and Forward

The method by which the medical images and data of patients are captured and stored locally in the TCC (telemedicine Consultation Centre) and/or at a central location n and subsequently forwarded/ transmitted to the TSC (telemedicine Specialty Center). In this method the Tele-consultation is carried out after the medical data is received at the TSC

Interoperability:

Develop Telemedicine networks that interface together and create an open environment sharing the application on different participating systems in real-time or seamless interface between several applications

Compatibility:

Equipment/ systems of different vendors and different versions of the same system, to be able to be interconnected.

Scalability:

Equipment/ systems inducted for Telemedicine to be able to be augmented with additional features and functions as modular add-on options.

Portability:

The data generated by an application that runs on one system to be able to be ported to different platforms with a minimum effort.

Reliability:

Tele-medicine systems to follow relevant reliability standards of equipment/systems of similar category to ensure availability of service with minimum system downtime.

Inclusion of all the stakeholders:

Making the recommendation with due consideration of the rights and responsibilities of patient/ community, health care service provider, the technology provider, the government etc.

Making recommendations vendor neutral:

Ensuring that the recommendations are not biased against any specific vendor/manufacturer of Telemedicine systems

Making standards technology neutral:

Ensuring that the recommendations will not favor any specific technology leaving scope for present/ future alternatives.

Unique Provider Identifiers

Unique Provider Identifiers in addition to overcoming communication and coordination difficulties, identifier would enhance the ability to eliminate fraud and abuse in health care programs -these include Unique Patient Identifier, Telemedicine centre identifier.

Unique Patient Identifier:

Each and every patient is identified by a unique and universal Patient Identifier. This Universal Patient Identifier will enable the benefits- Same patient can move across multiple providers without loss of data, one centralized PIR can be assimilated, Medical records database can be built and queried across time, Captures one-time patient demographics for later analysis.

Telemedicine Centre Identifier:

Each Telemedicine service center acting as either Telemedicine Consulting Centre (TCC) or Telemedicine Specialist Centre (TSC) or both is identified by a unique and universal identifier code. This Telemedicine Centre identifier -Allows for easy identification of provider for

Telemedicine purpose, only genuine hospitals can get onto Telemedicine network having proper infrastructure, allows for common billing format across providers, Registration number of providers can be used as identifier.

References:

1. Health Privacy Project at www.healthprivacy.org/info-url nocat2304info-url nocat.htm

2. HIPAA 101.com - Info Guide to HIPAA Compliance, Implementation and Privacy at www.hipaa-101.com

3. Computer Science and Telecommunications Board, Networking Health: Prescriptions for the Internet,2000.

4. Role Based Access Control at http://csrc.nist.gov/rbac

5. Serge Vaudenay, A Classical Introduction to Cryptography: Applications for Communications Security, Springer, 2006.

6. Meingast M, Roosta T, Sastry S, editors. Security and privacy issues with health care information technology. 2006 International Conference of the

IEEE Engineering in Medicine and Biology Society; 2006: IEEE.

7. *Dimitropoulos, L.L. (2007b) —Privacy and Security Solutions for Interoperable Health Information Exchange: Nationwide Summary, report for Agency for Healthcare Research and Quality, and Office of national Coordinator for Health Information Technology*

8. *Raghupathi, W., Kesh, S. (2007) —Interoperable Electronic Health Records Design: Towards a Service-oriented Architecture, e-Service Journal, pp. 39-57*

9. *Appari A, Eric Johnson M. Information security and privacy in healthcare: Current state of research12010. 279-314 p.*

10. *Harman LB, Flite CA, Bond KJAJoE. Electronic health records: Privacy, confidentiality, and security. 2012;14(9):712-9.*

11. *The AMA Code of Medical Ethics distinguishes confidentiality from privacy: AMA CODE OF ETHics E5.059.*

12. *WiLLIAM L. PROSsER, HANDBOOK OF THE LAW OF TORTS 802 (4th ed. 1971) (citing COOLEY, TORTS 29 (2d ed. 1888); Samuel D. Warren & Louis D. Brandeis, The Right to Privacy, 4 HARv. L. REv. 193 (1890)).*

13. *Lawrence Gostin et al., Privacy and Security of Health Information in the Emerging Health Care System, 5 HEALTH MATRIX 1, 21 (1995);*

14. *Anita L. Allen, Taking Liberties: Privacy, Private Choice, and Social Contract Theory, 56 U. CIN. L. REv. 461, 464 (1987)*

15. *Anita L. Allen, Coercing Privacy, 40 WM. & MARY L. REv. 723, 723-24 (1999); see Daniel J. Solove, Conceptualizing Privacy, 90 CAL. L. REv. 1087, 1092, 1116-18 (2002)*

16. *Gostin et al., supra note 22, at 3.*

17. *See Judy Zelin, Annotation, Physician's Tort Liability for Unauthorized Disclosure of Confidential Information About Patient, 48 A.L.R. 4TH 668, 679 (1986) 287 S.2d 824, 830-32 (1973)*

18. *Allen, supra note 22, at 464-65*

19. *Patient Confidentiality, Rayhan A. Tariq; Pamela B. Hackert, 2019, Book*

20. *Redefining the Health Information Management Privacy and Security Role, Laurie A. Rinehart-Thompson, JD, RHIA, CHP; Beth M. Hjort, RHIA, CHPS; and Bonnie S. Cassidy, MPA, RHIA, FAHIMA, FHIMSS, 2009*

21. *AHIMA*

22. *NHS*

23. *Ricardo Filipe Sousa Santos September, 2009*

24. *Kay, Misha, Jonathan Santos, and Marina Takane. "mHealth: New horizons for health through mobile technologies." World Health Organization 64.7 (2011): 66-71.*

31. *Challenges in implementing mHealth interventions: a technical perspective Varadraj P. Gurupur1 , Thomas T. H. Wan 2017*

32. *Extending the framework for Mobile Health Information Systems Research: A Content Analysis Shah Jahan Miah , John Gammack , Najmul Hasan*

33. *Methodological Review Mobile-health: A review of current state in 2015 Bruno M.C. Silva a,1 , Joel J.P.C. Rodrigues a,b, Isabel de la Torre Díez c,2 , Miguel López-Coronado c,2 , Kashif Saleem b,*

34. *Fatehi, Farhad, et al. "How to formulate research questions and design studies for telehealth assessment and evaluation."Journal of Telemedicine and Telecare (2016): 1357633X16673274.*

35. *Awareness and Use of mHealth Apps: A Study from England Reem Kayyali *, Aliki Peletidi, Muhammad Ismail, Zahra Hashim, Pedro Bandeira and Jennifer Bonnah 2017*

36. *Hum, A. P. 2001. Fabric area network - a new wireless communications infrastructure to enable ubiquitous networking and sensing intelligent clothing. Computer networks, 35(4), pp 391-399.*

37. *Zheng, Y. L., Ding, X. R., Poon, C. C. Y., Lo, B. P. L., Zhang, H., Zhou, X. L., Yang, G. Z., Zhao, N. & Zhang, Y. T. 2014. Unobtrusive sensing and wearable devices for health informatics. IEEE transactions on biomedical engineering, 61(5), pp 1538-1554.*

38. *Çiçek M. Wearable technologies and its future applications. International Journal of Electrical, Electronics and Data Communication. 2015;3:2320-084.*

39. *Massaroni, C., Saccomandi, P. & Schena, E. 2015. Medical smart textiles based on fibre optic technology: an overview. Journal of functional biomaterials, 6(2), pp 204-221.*

40. *Hänsel K, Wilde N, Haddadi H, Alomainy A. Challenges with current wearable technology in*

monitoring health data and providing positive behavioural support2015.